A FOREST BATHING
❧COMPANION❧

A FOREST BATHING ❧COMPANION❧

LEARN ABOUT NATURE'S REJUVENATING POWERS
ON A HEALING NATURE TRAIL WALK

TAMARACK SONG

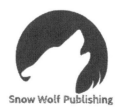

Snow Wolf Publishing

Snow Wolf Publishing
7124 Military Road
Three Lakes, Wisconsin 54562
www.snowwolfpublishing.org

Snow Wolf Publishing is a division of Teaching Drum Outdoor School

Song, Tamarack, 1948 –
The Healing Nature Trail: Forest Bathing for Recovery and Awakening

ISBN-13: 978-0-9894737-5-0
1. Forest Bathing 2. Natural Healing 3. Trauma Recovery

Text design and layout by James Arneson ~ JaadBookDesign.com

To send correspondence to the author of this book, mail a first class letter to the author c/o Snow Wolf Publishing, 7124 Military Road, Three Lakes, Wisconsin 54562, and we will forward the communication; or email the author at info@snowwolfpublishing.org.

Visit the author's websites at www.healingnaturecenter.org, www.teachingdrum.org, and www.snowwolfpublishing.org.

References to Internet websites (URLs) were accurate at the time of writing. Neither the authors nor Snow Wolf Publishing are responsible for URLs that may have expired or changed since this book was published.

Here is an introduction to Forest Bathing, as seen through the eyes of someone who is experiencing it for the first time. Whether you are being guided or going solo, and whether it's on a Healing Nature Trail or another pathway, this book prepares you for your restorative and re-awakening Nature-immersion experience. On these pages, you'll find grounding in many Nature-based therapies and ways to mindfully reconnect with Nature, along with a journey to self-discovery through Nature's guiding voices. The text is based on excerpts from *The Healing Nature Trail: Forest Bathing for Recovery and Awakening,* by Tamarack Song. Please see that book for comprehensive coverage of the health benefits, history, design, and management of Healing Nature Trails, along with extensive references and a description of Healing Nature Guide training.

Nothing can befall me in life—no disgrace, no calamity ... which nature cannot repair.

— **Ralph Waldo Emerson**

For Quick Reference

If you are stressed, grieving, or undergoing a major life change, go to page 127.

For the Trail map, go to page 18.

If you came to walk the Labyrinth, see page 21.

For general information on the Trail and personal preparation, go to page 6.

To learn more about how Nature heals, see page 91.

If you are a person with special needs, go directly to page 133.

For ways to support the Trail, see page 143.

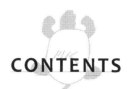

CONTENTS

CONTENTS

PART ONE

ONE PERSON'S EXPERIENCE: WALKING THE TRAIL WITH CHRIS AND HIS GUIDE, SARAH

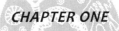

CHAPTER ONE

Why Chris Came, and What He First Finds

For most of his adult life, Chris has struggled with chronic stress and depression. It's been particularly rough since he broke up with his longtime girlfriend last year. He keeps playing the blame-shame game with himself. Even though he knows his travails are the legacy of childhood trauma—from an overly protective mother and an emotionally distant father—he can't seem to overcome it and get some traction in his life.

A few days ago, he came across this quote from Danish philosopher Søren Kierkegaard: "Above all, do not lose your desire to walk. Every day I walk myself into a state of well-being and walk away from every illness. I have walked myself into my best thoughts, and I know of no thought so burdensome that one cannot walk away from it." Those words gave Chris new hope. They express his reason for venturing into the farther places today, and what he hopes Nature in all her splendor will graciously provide him.

Chris first heard about the Healing Nature Trail from a friend. When Chris next saw his therapist, he mentioned the Trail to her, and she replied that she already knew about it as well. She encouraged him to go online and learn more about the Trail and Nature Therapy. There he found reference to numerous studies that showed how the sounds, smells, and visual effects of a captivating natural setting lead to reduced stress and support the healing process.

Now Chris would like to wander quietly and slowly down sylvan paths, taking in whatever appears around the next bend. With an open mind and senses enlivened, he wants to breathe in his surroundings and touch the soul of the life around him. The lilting birds, the many-hued flowers, the fragrant breeze in his face … He yearns for the gifts they have to share with him.

He came to the Trail today specifically to do that, because his therapist told him Healing Nature Trails provide uninterrupted quiet, security, and privacy, as they are reserved exclusively for use by people like him.

From reading the website, Chris remembers that he needs to pay attention as he comes up Military Road, as there is no sign to mark the turnoff to the Trail. There is only the address posted at the base of a nondescript driveway, which could pass for the entrance to any normal residence. The unpublished address (which he knows only because he preregistered), the inconspicuous entryway, and the fact that only registered users are allowed on the Trail, gives him the assurance of privacy and a sense of safety.

Yet there is one distinguishing feature that catches Chris's attention: the vibrant wildflower beds on either side of the entryway. An informative sign tells him that pollinators— particularly bees and butterflies—have been experiencing increased stress over the past decade. The loss of habitat due to agricultural practices, urbanization, climate change, and pesticides has caused a population crash, along with compromised health for the survivors.

Chris picks up a brochure from the holder below the sign, which describes how the Healing Nature Center staff engages in a mutual healing relationship with Nature by planting a wide variety of native wildflowers, as well as shrubs such as Staghorn Sumac (*Rhus typhina*) and Red Elderberry (*Sambucus racemosa*) to support pollinator species. An increase in pollinator habitat, says the brochure, leads directly to improved health and increased populations for bees and butterflies.

Reading on, Chris discovers that humans also benefit from the healing properties of floral essences and the aesthetics of blooming flowers being visited by hummingbirds and butterflies. Planting the beds is therapeutic in and of itself: it has a strong positive effect on mental and physical rehabilitation.

A warm feeling overcomes Chris as he recognizes the new flowerbeds and the butterflies it has attracted as a metaphor for the healing that could potentially manifest anywhere. Along with that, he is heartened by what the blooming flowers hint about his upcoming Trail experience.

The brochure states that, along with reintroducing wildflowers, the Healing Nature Center is actively engaged in reintroducing, protecting, and monitoring endangered and extirpated animal species, such as the Eastern Cottontail Rabbit (*Silvilagus floridanus*), Thirteen-Lined Ground Squirrel (*Letidomys tridecemlineatus*), Eastern Timber Wolf (*Canis lupus lycaon*), and various bird species. In addition, the Center has an invasive plant species eradication program. It focuses on non-toxic methods to control or eradicate alien plants that outcompete native species and disrupt the ecological balance.

Pulling up the drive, Chris sees the vehicle parking area immediately to the left, and on the right is a bicycle rack. There are picnic benches where he can sit and relax, and maybe have a snack while the nearby Gateway Labyrinth captures his attention.

But first Chris wants to refresh himself on what he can expect from the Trail. He reads in *The Forest Bathing Companion* that the main Trail is a half mile in length, with several side Trails forking off of it. The Trail, it says, is designed to bring him closer to Nature, which sometimes means direct physical and psychic contact. One way that's accomplished is by the Trail's soft, smooth surface, which is suitable for Barefoot Walking (also called *Earthing or Grounding,* as covered in chapter 8).

In *The Forest Bathing Companion*, Chris reviews the four main experiences he's been looking forward to:

- **Walking/Sitting Meditation.** The Guide says that the serene setting, with a Trail winding gently through stately

Pines, creates a classic setting for Walking Meditation. The gentle slopes, scenic overviews, and route options can have him spending from an hour to an afternoon in a deep meditative experience.

Rustic benches and the soft, carpeted forest floor under towering Elder Pines provide inviting private spaces for Sitting Meditation. In addition, nine off-Trail nooks overlooking expansive vistas rich with wildflowers and waterfowl can be reserved for solo and group meditation.

Everywhere, the book says, is the uplifting energy of Earth, Sky, and Water, along with the companionship of plant and animal kin. The Buddha asked us to join him by finding a tree to sit under, and here is a splendid opportunity to do so.

▶ **Day Retreats.** Chris has the option of spending a half or whole day out on a peninsula reserved just for him. Nestled in a sheltered grove of Spruce and Fir, he'll have a panoramic view of a classic Northwoods scene: a beaver pond and bog bordered by Pine and Birch.

▶ **Healing.** The Guide says that like all Healing Nature Trails, this one is designed for guided and self-guided healing immersions in Nature. Whether Chris comes alone or accompanied by a therapist or Healing Nature Guide, Nature is there to renew him.

▶ **The Labyrinthine Experience.** Many come just to Walk the Gateway Labyrinth or Zen Untangle, or to work in the Zen Garden (see chapter 6), says the Guide. The Cosmorinth (see chapter 9) is popular for evening visits. With each, Chris reads that there are choices to make, impasses to confront, and the opportunity to feel the connection between self and Nature. Or he might prefer a plate-size Finger Labyrinth, which allows him to travel the maze in whatever space calls him.

The Healing Power of Water

As Chris reads on, he is reminded that the Trail is located on an island Nature preserve, which is bordered by streams, ponds, and floating bog. The only easy access to the Trail is the Threshold Bridge, which helps to assure the privacy and integrity of the Trail experience.

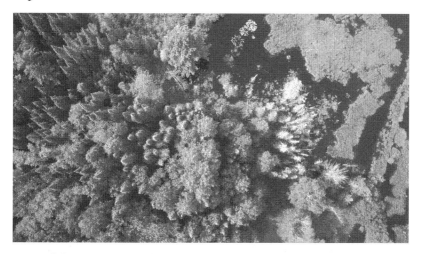

An Eagle's -eye view of the Sanctuary Island

The water theme is carried through in the island's interior, with the Trail skirting five ephemeral ponds. Here is an opportunity to view pond life up-close. In the spring and summer, frogs and turtles are busy tending to their affairs, while birds and dragonflies flit overhead. The Trail has been designed to keep Chris mostly in the shadows around the ponds, so he can observe without disturbing.

Water possesses tremendous healing power, which is one reason the Trail founders selected this site. Wetlands are Nature's filter, taking the runoff from the highlands and letting it percolate slowly through its dense mass of vegetation, where excess nutrients are taken up by the plants. The water then gets further purified as it filters down through the soil to recharge the water table.

When Chris visits a wetland, he can get taken in by this process, and it becomes a metaphor for his own cleansing and recharging. Water in itself has a calming effect. He remembers how refreshed he feels when he dangles his feet in the water of a lake or stream. Simply just splashing water on his face can center him and lift his spirits.

The therapeutic properties of water amplify the effect of other healing practices and explain why water plays a central role in many ceremonies. We see it in the Christian baptism and holy water anointing traditions, and in the water honoring and sweat lodge ceremonies of the Algonquin people of the Great Lakes Region (which is where the original Healing Nature Trail is located). The Trail staff feel deeply blessed to have the Mother Water, with her supportive healing properties, as such a central component of the Trail.

Trail Features

Reading further, Chris gains an overview of the therapeutic features of the Forest Pathways that fork and rejoin as they meander across wetlands, around ponds, over ridges, and through groves of Elder Trees:

- **Conifer Bough Smudge**: for cleansing before setting foot on the Trail.
- **Remembering Cairn**: for making an intention and placing an offering before his Walk, then taking a memento after.
- **Threshold Bridge**: leave all baggage, cross the arch to enter the island preserve and trailhead on the other side, and immerse in the trusting embrace of Uncharted Nature.
- **Numerous Foot Bridges:** encourage fresh perspective.
- **Two Meeting Circles**: located in the Pines, with one having a Ceremonial Fire Pit.
- **Log Benches beside the Trail**: nestled between pairs of Elder Pines.

▶ **Eight Labyrinths:** the Gateway Labyrinth with wild-flower-bordered Paths, Cosmorinth, Stump Labyrinth, Aquarinth, Finger Labyrinths, Zen Untangle, and Zen Garden. And the Trail itself functions as a Labyrinth when one stays on the main Pathways.

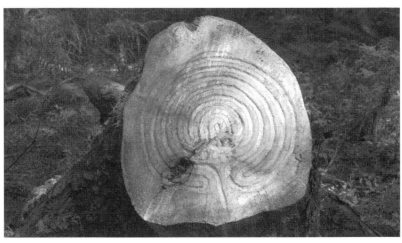

The Stump Labyrinth, which is patterned after the Gateway Labyrinth

▶ **Nine Private Nooks:** for reflection, Sitting Meditation, and one-on-one therapeutic work.

▶ **The Water Therapy Beaver Dam:** for Water Grounding and bathing in negative ions generated by tumbling water.

▶ **Three Side-Trail Loops:** serve as metaphors for the choices we face on our Healing Journey.

▶ **No Informative Signs:** language is a strictly rational process, which detracts from engaging in the awakening and deep-healing work that falls in the realm of the limbic system—the seat of emotions, long-term memories, and intuition.

▶ **Special Trail Access Features:** for the physically and developmentally challenged.

Regarding the last point, Chris noticed when he parked his car that next to him was a space reserved for Trail users in wheelchairs. From that spot, he saw a separate wheelchair-friendly Trail crossing a threshold bridge spanning the nearby pond, then meandering through the adjacent meadow of prairie wildflowers and into a Pine grove.

A Place of Reverence

Lastly, just before Chris goes to register at the Welcome Center, he reads that over the years people have requested that their ashes, or the ashes of loved ones, be spread along the Healing Nature Trail. The *Forest Bathing Companion* and *Healing Nature Trail* books state that most Trails are located in Nature preserves, where final remains can lie undisturbed, and where they can be visited in peace.

Some saw having their ashes spread along the Trail as their final Healing Walk. They wanted to rest in the presence of others who, like them, came to abide in Nature's comfort. The parents of a child who died an untimely death wanted his last resting place to be on sacred ground, where he would become a part of something they felt good about. Another person wanted to return to the original mother who bore him—to Nature—when he died. In the ultimate sense, he saw his nature as Nature.

The Huitil Maya of Central America share that perspective. They see both birth and death being midwifed, with us not releasing our loved ones, but helping them echo on through the soil, wildflowers, and animals, as well as the nourishing water and cleansing wind.

Knowing this, many people Walk the Trail with a sense of reverence. The awareness that they stand in the presence of others who have come before them empowers their Healing and Awakening Journeys.

Checking In at the Welcome Center

Chris already decides to leave his watch and handheld device behind, so he can immerse himself in the Trail experience without distraction. To lose time is to become the moment and merge with the surroundings, and that's one of the reasons he came. Yet now he wants to make sure the Welcome Center is open so he can register. He checks the posted times on the Center door:

> **TRAIL AND LABYRINTH USE**
> **BY RESERVATION ONLY.**
>
> **Summer hours: 8:00 AM to 6:00 PM**
> **Tue.- Sun. May 15 - October 15**
>
> **Evening Cosmorinth use by appointment**
> **Winter hours: by appointment.**
>
> **For service call 715-546-8080**

Before Chris enters, however, he gets distracted by the birch-bark and thatch-covered wigwams that catch his eye under a large, spreading Pine at the far side of the Cosmorinth. He recognizes it as the type of lodge once used by the Northern Woodland Natives, and it makes him wonder about the region's heritage and ecology, and how the Trail fits in. He's now all the more looking forward to touring the Trail History Museum, which he plans to do after he registers for the Trail Walk.

Check-In and Trail Fees

Right away, Chris is surprised that there is no set charge for Trail usage. He is informed that the policy is based on the shamanic healing principle that giving is receiving. Nature is the healer, so the fewer requirements placed upon Trail users, the easier it is for Trail staff to step aside and let Nature do her work.

Setting a fee can create an expectation, which if not met could create resentment. Such a mercenary edge might interfere with the body-mind connection. Being open and welcoming, with as few prerequisites as possible, fosters a sense of openness and feeling of trust, both of which are highly conducive to listening and receiving.

Chris is told that whatever he feels inclined to contribute after he completes his Walk is acceptable.

Yet there are some people who do not feel comfortable operating under this premise. They either want to contribute up front or if they wait until the completion of their Walk, they want a solid suggestion for what to contribute. For them, forcing an unfamiliar protocol could cause more harm than good, so the Welcome Center staff suggests a contribution amount.

Trail usage contributions are separate from Healing Nature Guide or therapist fees. Guides and healthcare practitioners enter into their own contractual relationships with their clients.

Special Services

Certified Healing Nature Guides are available to take Chris on the Trail. They would help him get the most from his Trail experience. As professionals with extensive training, they know the Trail and its features well, and they have guided many people. They have been vetted and trained to follow ethical guidelines, so Chris can feel safe with them. Healing Nature Guides have also received special training to guide people with visual impairments and clients in wheelchairs (see chapter 14).

Since this is his first time on the Trail, Chris wants to get the most out of the experience, so he decides to go with a Guide. Her name is Sarah, and she has already given him an overview of what to expect and answered his questions regarding registration. The two of them decide that it would be best for him to experience the preparatory process of the Gateway Labyrinth, Smudge, Cairn, and Threshold Bridge on his own. Quoting Deepak Chopra, that "solitude is the great teacher, and to learn its lessons you must pay attention to it," Sarah adds that she's glad Chris is starting his Walk alone. She will wait for him on Breathing Knoll, which is the first stop on the Trail.

But first Sarah will conduct a Conscious Walking Workshop (see chapter 6) for him and a couple other Trail Walkers who are being guided by their therapists. Chris planned his arrival to coincide with the workshop, as he's learned through his Walking Meditation practice that Conscious Walking is a great way for him to bring his total being into a state of conscious presence.

Clothing and Gear

The Welcome Center staff person gives Chris a weather report and checks to make sure he is appropriately outfitted for the day and Trail conditions. The general recommendations for how to dress and what to bring are:

- **Lightweight Clothing.** Weather permitting, wear clothing that exposes some skin to the air and sun, and allows some bare-skin contact with the ground and plants.
- **An Extra Layer** of seasonally appropriate clothing, including raingear.
- **Footwear.** Wear light, flexible footwear, without rubber soles if possible, to allow for maximum contact with the ground. Moccasins are ideal.
- **Insect Repellent** in spring and summer.
- **Sun Protection,** sunscreen and/or a wide-brimmed hat and protective clothing.
- **Notebook** and art supplies (for art therapy and nonverbal expression).
- **Water.** Bring only water on the Trail, as the flavors and odors of other beverages can interfere with the healing essences of the Earth and the Trees.
- **Food.** A snack for the Trail, and something for the Trail's End Feast of Gratitude (as mentioned in chapter 7).
- **Small Backpack or Shoulder Bag,** to comfortably carry everything.

Trail Tokens

For some people, Tokens are valued—even necessary—companions on significant steps of their Life Journeys. For others, it may be time to set old and familiar supports aside in order to venture forth with a fresh sense of trust and openness. When we hold onto something, it can be hard to fully experience free flight. As helpful as our traveling companions have been, we sometimes need new voices and fresh inspiration.

On his initial call, a staff person encouraged Chris to bring a Crystal, Feather, Stuffed Animal, Picture, Keepsake ... any Token that he typically carried for empowerment, comfort, or security. He was told that Tokens could be left at the Trailhead Remembering Cairn (see chapter 3), then picked up when he completed his Walk. Or he may come to realize that it is his time to fly, and he decides to leave his Token at the Cairn for someone else. Other Tokens he wants to be held securely or that are weather-sensitive can be left at the Welcome Center, to be reclaimed after his Walk.

Chris typically shies away from what he considers to be primitive practices, but the Tokens up on the top shelf catch his eye. He sees Bear, Turtle, Fox, Eagle, Dolphin, and Frog Tokens, among others, carved from wood and stone. He's also drawn to the brightly colored, fanciful creatures that the staff person calls *Alebrije* Tokens. Trail cofounder Lety Siebel is from the indigenous Oaxacan culture of southern Mexico where Alebrijes originated, and she has introduced the mystical Alebrije Tokens to many people.

Next to the Alebrijes sits a similar hybrid animal that possesses aquatic and terrestrial features. She is a *Hodag*, the contemporary incarnation of the ancient Spirit-Keeper of the Northcountry Waters.

The Token who originally drew Chris's attention speaks to him, and for some unexplainable reason, he is not surprised. The staff person hands it to Chris, who reverently tucks it into the breast pocket over his heart. (More on Tokens in chapter 11.)

A Gifting Shop

As an afterthought, Chris asks how much the Token costs. The attendant hands it to him so caringly that it seemed to be a sharing from the heart rather than a transaction, which made him momentarily forget his assumption that the items displayed in the Welcoming Center must be for sale. Yet as he looks around, he sees that most items are not priced.

"Nearly everyone is confused at first," explains the attendant. "But just like ours is no ordinary Nature trail, this isn't the type of gift shop people typically expect. It's more like a *gifting* shop, as nearly everything that's Trail related—Tokens, Finger Labyrinths, Drums, Rattles, art supplies—is available for use at no charge."

"But what if I want to take the Token home with me?" Chris replies.

"That's possible, and you can leave a donation for it to cover the Center's cost. If you need a suggested donation amount, we can do that. Yet the real value of something like a Token or Finger Labyrinth (a plate-size portable Labyrinth) goes beyond its monetary value—it comes from the many hands that have caringly held her and the awarenesses and healings she has witnessed. It's like an antique, with a patina and an intrinsic value that no reproduction can match."

Welcome Center Stock Items

For Trail Use

▶ **Trail Maps**

▶ **Handouts** on Conscious Breathing, Labyrinth therapy, Trail Meditations, pollinator restoration, and others

▶ **Moccasins**

▶ **Paddles and Lifejackets** for the Aquarinth

▶ **Drums**, Rattles, and Rainsticks

▶ **Sitting Pads,** basic and sheepskin, for use on the Trail

- **Finger Labyrinths** in three styles
- **Art Supplies:** colored pencils, crayons, charcoal, and sketch pads
- **Tokens** of Animal Guides, Crystals or Feathers
- **Backpacks and Shoulder Bags**

Also available

- **T-shirts** and hoodies with Trail and Labyrinth logos
- **Notebooks**
- **Insect Repellent and Headnets**
- **Aromatherapy Essential Oils** from trees found on the Trail
- **Books** on awakening to Nature, Labyrinths, Zen, trauma, emotional healing, and two books on the Healing Nature Trail
- **Traditional Birchbark Baskets**
- **Notecards** by the late Ojibwe artist Moses (Amik) Beaver
- **Gift Certificates**

The Final Preparation

"There's one more thing I'd like to mention," says the staff person. "You've probably heard that curiosity killed the Cat; but you may not know the rest of the saying—that satisfaction brought her back. The same is true for us when we embrace our fear and let it be our guide to awakening and healing. When fear controls us, we cannot open up enough to trust and listen."

"Then why do I hang on to fear?" asks Chris.

"Some of us dread what is inside of us, and some of us are concerned that others will control us. The irony is that we are already controlled by our fear. Yet without fear to guide us, we are not ready to heal. As Indian mystic Osho said, "Courage is a love affair with the unknown—a love affair with fear." Courage is nothing more than fear-infused curiosity, and this is what we need in order to be a trailblazer into our healing frontier.

"Without fear, there are no love affairs—no love for the life we want to heal, and no love for our Mother Nature who wants to help heal us. And let's not forget that love affairs are fun. The Healing Journey is an adventure, and healing makes us feel good. In the deepest sense, fear is fun in disguise. Why else would the Cat keep dancing out on her edge?"

Chris packs up what he's taking with him on his Walk, and he's ready to go. The staff person asks that he take all trash out with him, including food scraps. Wishing him a fulfilling Walk, she adds that he should have uninterrupted one-on-one time with Nature, as no more than ten people are allowed on the Trail at any one time.

"Plan on about two hours for a basic Trail Walk," she tells Chris. "Of course with the Gateway Labyrinth and any other features you take advantage of, you could easily double or triple that time.

"By the way," she adds, "did you grab a Trail Meditations handout from the shelf here (see chapter 8)? You may not need it, but I suggest taking one anyway, just in case you hit a flat spot and need some inspiration."

As Chris steps outside, he orients himself by looking at the foldout Trail map he just picked up in the Welcome Center. Getting the full picture of the Trail layout, he catches his breath as he suddenly realizes that the Trail is a mosaic of the mind—and that he is about to take a metaphorical Journey into its inner realms! There it is: the Trail's folds and forks make it look like a giant Labyrinth, and he remembers reading that Labyrinths may be patterned after the many-folded appearance of the brain.

Taking a calming breath, Chris heads over to meet Sarah and the others for the Conscious Walking Workshop, then to begin his Nature immersion at the Gateway Labyrinth.

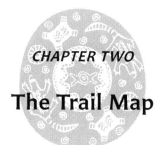

CHAPTER TWO

The Trail Map

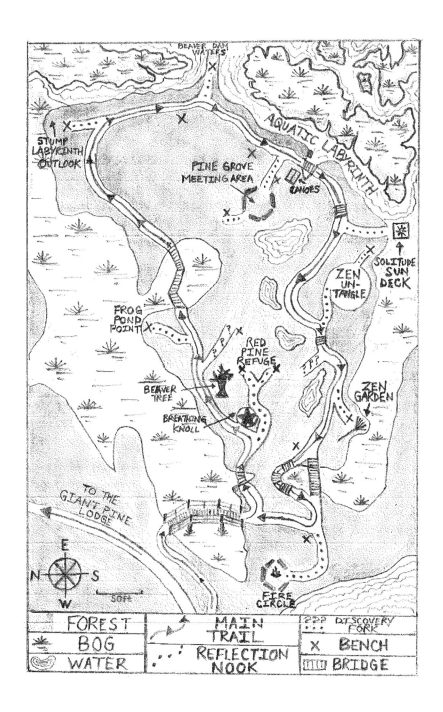

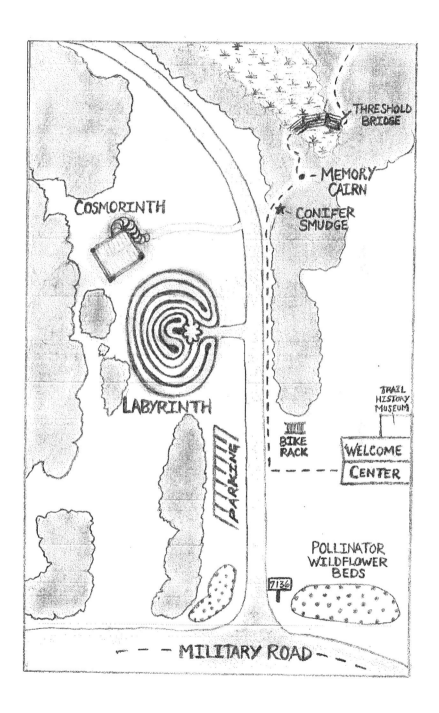

CHAPTER THREE

Unwind at the Labyrinths

Whether someone is being accompanied by a Certified Healing Nature Guide, their healthcare practitioner, or this text, it is recommended that they begin their Walk here at one of the Trail Gateway Labyrinths. By day, the gateway is our classic Labyrinth, inspired by the design found throughout ancient Babylon, Egypt, Persia, and Greece. The Labyrinth's Path is bordered by multicolored wildflowers, who support declining Bee and Butterfly populations. In the evening, the Cosmorinth is the gateway to the Labyrinthine Journey amongst the planets and constellations.

The Labyrinth is a special type of maze, designed to help unwind the body and quiet the mind. Comprised of a single Path that coils in from the perimeter starting point to its center, a Labyrinth guides one back out on the same Path.

As opposed to standard mazes, there are no forks in a Labyrinth's Path and no dead ends. With no decisions to make, one has the opportunity to give herself completely over to the experience. All she has to do is follow the Path, and she is guaranteed to reach the center and return to where she started.

There is one more thing: she must be present. The Labyrinth gives no other choice, because its Path twists and turns to the right and left, doubling back upon itself numerous times as it takes her deeper and deeper toward the center. The return Path is the same, only in reverse.

The only choice she has to make is how present she wants to be. The more she engages her senses of sight, smell, and hearing, the more present she will be, and the more she will gain from the experience.

One beauty of the Labyrinthine Experience is that being present is all one has to do—the Labyrinth does the rest.

As the Labyrinth guides her, a sense of trust and safety, of being cradled, will permeate her being. The tensions and concerns that she brought with her, and the drama of the wild world she lives in, seem to dissipate as though they were many layers of a heavy overcoat on a hot day. A sense of peace comes over her, leaving her in the state of conscious being, with uncluttered space for listening.

The Gateway by Day: A Classic Turf Labyrinth

The Labyrinth lies in the middle of a grassy meadow at the beginning of the Healing Nature Trail. Bordered by a pond and surrounded by towering pines, the site itself is calming and inviting.

A short stone-lined Path across the driveway from the Welcome Center takes Chris to the threshold of the Labyrinth. At the beginning of the Path he notices a Cairn of many-spangled stones, with a sign beside it that reads:

> **One left**
> **for an Offering**
> **One to**
> **accompany your Walk**
> **One to**
> **take for remembrance**

Chris caringly tucks the Crystal who asked to come along with him into his pocket as he slowly travels down the Path. Looking ahead, he takes in the sheer majesty of the ancient-looking panorama laid out before him.

The Journey Inward

Chris enters the Labyrinth from the South, the direction of nourishment and support. As he steps over the threshold, he realizes right away that he has entered a living organism. The Path is carpeted with soft grasses, and the Path's borders are festooned with herbs and flowers. Chris is infused with life-energy—he can feel it, smell it, and hear it.

After only a few paces, he skirts the edge of the Labyrinth's heart—a small grotto in the shape of a six-petaled flower. The center design is inspired by that of the Chartres Cathedral in France, which is laid out in mosaic tile on the cathedral floor.

The design parallels the Seven-Direction cosmology of the Algonquian people of eastern North America. Along with the four cardinal directions (South for nourishment, West for wisdom, North for introspection, and East for new beginnings), there is the Above, the Below, and the Within.

Yet the grotto has only six petals. The seventh is the stem of the flower: the Path that leads into the grotto from the East. The Algonquians keep an opening on the eastern side of ceremonial circles to allow for the easy entry of inspiration and fresh starts. However, it is not yet Chris's time to immerse in the Heart of the Journey. As close as he is, he is still separated from it by a hedge. The Labyrinth's intention is to inspire him by giving him only a hint of what is to come.

After briefly skirting the Heart, the Path veers off and loses itself in a web of its own making. From above, the pattern looks, not coincidentally, like the folds of a brain.

The Trail now takes Chris in a wide clockwise arc around the entire Labyrinth about midway between the Heart and the perimeter. He ends up back near the entrance, to be reminded about where he began and what brought him here.

Yet he is not here to linger, as the Trail doubles back upon itself and takes him all the way back around the Labyrinth, to the opposite side of the entrance. Here again, he is reminded why he came and to whence he shall return, which helps him maintain perspective and gives him the motivation to continue. Again, he doubles back, this time skirting the very outer edge of the serpentine form. He is able to gaze out over the perimeter hedge and drink in the undulating waves of meadow herbs and flowers, pristine and undisturbed. The serenity, the taste of what could be, accompanies Chris all the way around the Labyrinth's perimeter, until he comes for the third time right up to the entryway.

However, this time the Path turns to take him deeply into the bowels of the Labyrinth, the dark recesses of his soul. On the way in, he again skirts the Heart, to be given another taste of what he may reach.

Yet he does not stay long, as the Path turns his back to the Heart, only to spin him back around and have him travel straight onto it and stare into its depths. There he lingers, feeling the draw to his Journey's fulfillment.

No, it is not yet the time. The Path whisks him off to the north, in the opposite direction of the heart, only to befuddle him by doubling back and taking him quickly right back to the Heart's edge. This time his sojourn with the Heart is *very* brief, and he again descends into the darkness of his undifferentiated inner landscape.

Back and forth Chris goes, through tight, dizzying turns, until—as though it were a mirage appearing before him—the Heart-Center sits at his feet. He steps into it and feels the flush of accomplishment, along with a sense of finality and release.

The Heart is a place for Chris to linger, to drink the nectar that is beaded up on each Heart-petal, with its unique and empowering gifts for the Return Journey.

The Way Back

Enriched blood lingers not long in Chris's heart. It is a vibrant organ, with a strong sense of ultimate purpose: to send him back on his Return Journey, to retrace his steps, imprinting in his memory all that he has gained on this quest, so that he may take it back and transform his life.

On the way back, Chris erases what he has shed on the way in, like fresh blood scouring the plaque that has accumulated on artery walls. He has come in on this arterial Path from the extended limbs of his life, into his core—his Heart-of-Hearts—to regain what he has lost touch with.

Now Chris is sent back to those outer reaches of his personal universe. Cleansed and empowered, he feels lighter on the way out. Still, each step is conscious, as he remembers what he has come here to forget. He does not want to lose a single teaching, a single reminder of what he brought with him and why he had to experience it. In this way, his travails become his teachings, his blockages become his open windows, and his blindness takes him to breathtaking vistas.

As some people leave the Labyrinth, they may be overtaken by laughter or tears; or they could be either overwhelmed or numbed-out. Chris is surprised at the deep peace that has descended upon him. Yet the state of being does not matter, as it is merely a passing cloud on these first steps of the new and unfolding Labyrinthine Path of our Life.

The Night and Day Gateway: The Cosmorinth

After Walking the Labyrinth, Chris notices the elevated platform with the spiral staircase off to the far right. Now he wants to experience it, so he approaches the serpentine stone-lined Pathway leading up to its spiral staircase.

Yet before he sets foot on the Path, Chris notices a Cairn similar to the one at the head of the Path to the Labyrinth. Only this one seems more bejeweled. He looks closely, and he sees Crystals of myriad shapes, forms, and hues. He reads the little sign at the base of the Cairn and picks up a Crystal that feels warm to the touch.

> **A Crystal in your hand**
> **Crystals in the sky**
> **Let the one you hold**
> **Help your spirit fly**

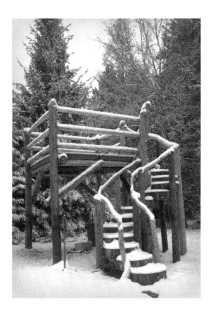

The closer Chris gets to the structure, the more it appears to have emerged from the surrounding Forest. The platform, which looks to be eight or ten feet wide and deep, perches atop four weathered tree trunks. Winding around one of the trunks is a staircase made from a massive log cut into roughly eight-inch thick discs, then stacked to form the steps. The railing, crafted from gnarled and twisted tree branches, seems like it grew right there to meet the need.

Before ascending the staircase, Chris reads the placard mounted off to one side:

Inspired by the shipbuilding tradition of placing a gold coin beneath the mast before it is raised, symbolic stones have been placed beneath the Cosmorinth's primary pillar: the one supporting this staircase. In shipbuilding, the gesture was done with the intention of making the ship's voyages safe and fruitful. The intention here is the same, for the cosmic voyage you are about to embark upon.

Here are the stones resting under the mast:

Meteorite *is the remnant of an asteroid or comet that has survived the intense heat and speed of crashing through Earth's atmosphere. The placement of a Meteorite under the foundational pillar gives cosmic presence to the viewing platform, as well as a reminder of the infinite possibilities of the universe.*

Tektite, *composed of silica, is formed when large comets or asteroids crash into the Earth. The tremendous force of impact causes terrestrial rock to melt and get thrown into the atmosphere. The lava-like spray, transformed into Tektite, falls back to Earth. As offspring of both Earth and Sky, just as we are, they symbolize our Cosmorinthine Journey: coming from Earth, venturing into the Sky, transforming, then returning to Earth.*

Moqui Stones, *also known as Shaman's Marbles, are concretions of sandstone encased in iron oxide. In Hopi legend, the ancestors use these stones to play marble games. When finished, the ancestors let their marbles lay, to tell their living relations they are happy. The Moqui Stone symbolizes our past-present-future connection, and it serves as a reminder that healing from yesterday, in order to experience a better tomorrow, begins today.*

Daytime Use

Chris, like nearly everyone else, first partakes of the breathtaking view of the Labyrinth from this high vantage point. Then he notices the telescope, which is used at night for intimate Journeying amongst the celestial orbs.

Right now though, Chris is more drawn to the cushioned seating, which he arranges so that he can lay down comfortably and let his gaze drift into the infinite. Today there is a sky of broken clouds, bordered by ever-changing azure Pathways. He takes several deep, relaxing breaths, then melds into the Labyrinthine Skyscape, which has no boundaries and infinite possibilities. There are the meandering Pathways in the treetops, and the trails taken by overhead Birds and Butterflies. And on a cloudless day like this, one can lose himself in the vast expanse of the blue, blue sky.

On his way down the spiral staircase, Chris notices another daytime user: the Bees who nest in the log's wormholes. With the nectar and pollen provided by the wildflowers in the beds the Center has established, along with the nesting habitat provided by the Center, there has been a sizable increase in the Bee and Butterfly populations.

FOR MEDITATION

Day or night, several people are so enamored with meditating suspended between Earth and Sky that they come regularly to sit. Some incorporate conscious sky gazing into their practices, and others blindfold themselves, to travel their inner Cosmos.

Journey into the Night

As beautifully as the Cosmorinth serves by day, it takes on an entirely different persona by night. The world below disappears, and the world above comes alive. All is cool and quiet, and there are no distractions. Sensory input is cut to a minimum. One can hear his breathing; one can hear his heartbeat.

For those reasons, many people prefer coming in the evening rather than the daytime. If someone arrives early enough, he can partake in a Sunset Smudge atop the Cosmorinth. Being cleansed by the last of the sun's golden rays, he will be uplifted by cosmic energy and ready for his upcoming amble through the Celestial

Maze. Chris plans on staying overnight at the Healing Nature Center's Giant Pine Lodge, so that he can also experience the Cosmorinth's nighttime magic.

There is no lighting on the Path to the Cosmorinth, or on its steps or viewing platform. Someone who arrives after dark is given a small red-lens flashlight to find his way. Red light barely disrupts the nighttime calm, as most animals cannot see red light, and the dull hue is only minimally disturbing to humans. A guest is asked to turn his light off as soon as he gets situated on the platform.

In the Celtic Druid tradition, the night sky is seen as a Crystal Cavern. It is entered on a solo Journey to discover what treasures for the psyche lie amongst the countless Crystals bejeweling the cavern.

Dusk is the threshold bridge a person crosses, from the brightness and business of his everyday life to the indefinable realm of the boundless interior. He passes over from the sure to the unsure, from the tenuous comfort of distractions and escapes to the uneasy awareness that soon there will be nowhere to turn but inward. There is nothing left other than his shaky grip on what he thought he had.

Without form or direction, he drifts aimlessly around the Great Cosmic Maze. He tries to gain some footing on the undulating Pathways of the Northern Lights, but they defy his intent and keep dancing to a different drum.

Other nights, it could be the skeletons of trees silhouetted by the rising Moon; or the ever-unfolding patterns of clouds across the Moon and Stars; or the craters, ridges, and plains of the lunar landscape, expanded across the sky by the Cosmorinth's telescope.

Any of these Labyrinths embedded within the Cosmic Cavern can fling him into the void of Outer-Inner Space. Once there, he comes to know what baggage he carried with him, because he cannot shake free of its grasp. If it burns to the touch, he knows without a doubt that it is something he needs to heal through. The real beginning of the Healing Journey is when he has no choice but to take full responsibility for what he holds in his grasp. It can only be his, because he drifts alone with it through the Cosmos. There is no one around to blame, and no one to rescue him.

This is the gift of the night. This is what he came for: just him and the ultimate Labyrinth—the Cosmos. Here he has the quint-essential, all-encompassing yin and yang: The Cosmic Inferno. And within that, Cosmic Harmony.

Some people like to think that when crossing the threshold of dusk and being swallowed into the night, they leave everything they know behind. The stark reality is just the opposite, as is often the case with what one thinks he knows. All that gets shed is what he assumes to know, or what he hopes to someday know, or what he was told is important to know but was never quite able to grasp.

What he truly knows is what remains in the deep, dark silence when all else is stripped away. This is all he takes with him—this is all he *can* take with him—when he tumbles into the galactic freefall known as the Cosmorinthine Journey.

Chris is now fully prepared. He is centered, stripped of excess bag-gage, and has a vision to fulfill on his upcoming Walk. The Forest looms ahead, and he is filled with anticipation. Yet he knows from hard experience that the joy of discovery carries with it the agony of knowing. If ignorance is not always bliss, then at least it makes few demands.

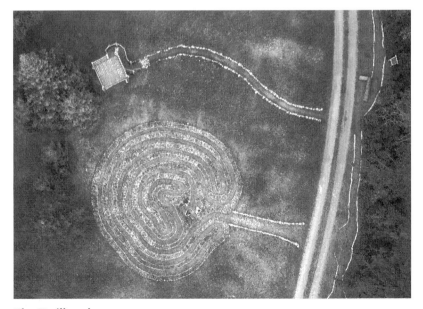

CHAPTER FOUR

Chris's First Steps

Chris is about to enter the maze called the Healing Nature Trail. Unlike the Labyrinth, this maze is a complex of Pathways without a clear route to the center. There are false starts and dead-ends, and—as with many of life's decisions—Chris may have to retrace his steps to get back on track … or at least what he thinks is on track.

Yet two things are certain: he will have to take personal responsibility for his venture, and he will have to risk going out

The Trailhead

on his edge. There is no guarantee that he will make it through the maze. Nor is it clear that he has to make it through in order to reach his goal.

Nowhere is "Nothing ventured, nothing gained," more true than here. With the maze, the courage to venture forth is the courage to heal. That means extending trust—not in any particular person or belief or healing modality, but rather trust in the process. When there is movement, there is the potential for change. And when the movement is conscious, the maze becomes a passageway to the mysteries of the mind and the knowing of the heart.

Chris's optimism wanes. The Labyrinth just took him on a Journey to the center of his mind, where he found a morsel of inner peace and self-knowing—a moment of hope. Yet now he feels defeated before he starts. Time and again he has struggled mightily to make it through that maze to the treasures of the mind and heart. Every time though, he ends up on his knees, whimpering. With every passageway he tries, he keeps hitting dead ends made up of the boundaries between his heart and mind. He knows that the longest Walk before him today is not the Trail itself, but rather the distance between his heart and mind— that's the Wolf in his belly.

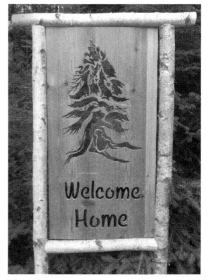

He drags his feet to the trail-head, which is directly across from the Labyrinth. He steps foot on the Trail, looks up, and his eyes meet this sign (see right):

The image sends a chill up his spine. "That's why I'm here!" he exclaims. In that instant, it comes clear that his appointment was not with the Center, but with his destiny.

The Gateway Sign

Then he reads the words below the image: *Welcome home,* and a tear finds its way down his cheek.

The small sign on the wall in the Welcome Center that read "Leave your baggage here" now makes sense to him. Thanks to the Labyrinth, he's been able to release his grip on much of what would otherwise have kept his mind someplace else, even though he is physically here. Another sign on the wall: "The lighter your load, the easier your Walk," takes on additional meaning.

Under the trailhead sign is a log bench, which reminds Chris of one more thing he wanted to do to lighten his load and ease his Walk. He sits down to remove his shoes and socks, so that he can take full advantage of the restorative benefits of Grounding (see chapter 8). Chris could have borrowed a pair of light moccasins from the Welcoming Center—which he was tempted to do because he is not accustomed to going barefoot—but he reads that the maintenance crew Walks the Trail barefoot every morning to make sure it's comfortable, and he trusts in that.

The Trailhead Smudge

No glance ahead can give Chris a clue to what is coming, as the Trail quickly disappears into the Pines. He sets foot on the Path, and he notices that, with every step, it narrows. The grove of young conifers that the Trail cuts through is closing in on either side, to the point that boughs are brushing his clothing and bare skin.

Shouldn't the vegetation have been trimmed back, Chris wonders. *Is the whole Trail going to be like this?*

Then he smells the piney fragrance of the boughs. It's pleasant, and it lifts his spirits. "Ah," he says to himself, "this is the Conifer Smudge I read about. No wonder I'm feeling good!"

The essence causes Chris to remember also reading that here and there throughout the Trail, branches, ferns, and sedges will caress him; and that they get cut back only when absolutely necessary, to maintain the Smudge effect. A warm smile graces his face.

The book went on to state that Smudging is a traditional practice akin to burning incense, anointing with holy water or essential oil, or the washing of feet or hands that often precedes ceremonies. Here in the forest, the cleansing essences come raw from the plants—a living Smudge—rather than being released by burning or extraction. Yet the effect is the same: the feeling of being cleansed and refreshed, and the pheromone-like properties transpose one to another state of consciousness. Some very psychic-sensitive people can be sent into a trance state from a Smudge alone.

Potawatomi elder and college professor Robin Wall Kimmerer is quoted in the book as saying that "ceremonial smudge … washes the recipient in kindness and compassion to heal the body and spirit."

So prepared, Chris ventures onward.

THE BRUSH-DOWN SMUDGE

For people who are suffering a high state of anxiety or are heavily traumatized, a vigorous Smudge is often necessary. Their therapist or Trail Guide will take a fan of boughs in each hand, have them take off their hats and glasses, and brush them down all around, from head to foot.

First Stop: The Remembering Cairn

A few steps beyond the Conifer Smudge, Chris comes to a small, neatly stacked pile of multicolored stones and unique pieces of driftwood. He brought a stone along—a special one given to him by a lover who left him in pain. He's never been able to come to peace with that relationship, and now he wants to release his attachment.

Chris gently places the stone on the backside of the Cairn, so he won't have to look at it again. That should make it easier, he thinks, but tears still flow.

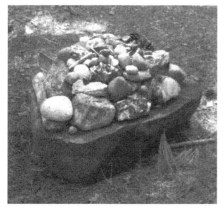

The Remembering Cairn

To fill the void, Chris chooses another stone with a shape and color different than his lover's gift. But then he puts it back, realizing that a substitution alone will not erase the pain. Instead, he chooses to Walk the Trail alone. He wants to come alive again: he wants to feel the pain, because he knows that if he doesn't allow it, he won't be able to feel himself.

Chris has come to find out who he is, and he is now ready to venture forth, alone and apprehensive. He thinks that maybe on the way back he will stop here and see if he is ready to take another stone home with him, to mark the memory of his newfound relationship with his rediscovered self.

Crossing the Threshold Bridge

Back on the Trail, Chris immediately enters a grove of tall Balsam Firs. Just as quickly, he takes a left turn, then a right, and finds

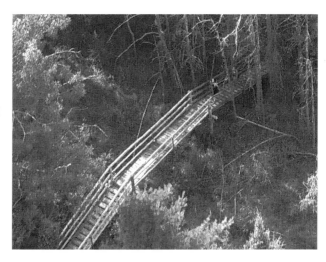

The Threshold Bridge

himself at the foot of a rustic wooden bridge. It's a long span, and he sees that it arches over an expanse of wetland.

Chris can't make out what's on the other side, and he knows he's not supposed to. He trusts that the shadowy Forest will accept and guide him when he is ready. But first he knows that he must face his threshold—this bridge between things he has trouble letting go of and things he may have trouble hearing.

This is Chris's last opportunity to either turn back or commit himself fully to his Healing Journey. There is nothing in between but the all-consuming Bog. She does not discriminate: whoever lingers indecisively breaks through the floating mat of vegetation and becomes hopelessly mired in regret and defeatism.

The lure to bridge the Bog is there: the song of birds and tall pines swaying lazily in the breeze beckon Chris. Yet the stronger the draw, the tighter his chest constricts.

One reason is that he can still pick up on the subtle sights and sounds of civilization behind him. Even though he read in the Trail literature that a last reminder of what he is leaving behind could help give him clarity on why he is here, he still wishes that distraction wasn't here at this critical moment.

Taking a deep, clearing breath, Chris tells himself it's now or never. He places one foot on the first wooden slat. His courage builds, and his other foot follows. It has now become the Bridge of No Return.

Only the slope is steep. Chris grabs the handrail to help him along. *Yes, I will need help,* he reminds himself. *I need help now. I know the Caring Mother awaits, and I know her plant and animal children are there to support and guide me. I just have to release myself—at least for this day—from the made-up beliefs that have been blinding me and the numbing crutches I have been leaning on.*

Chris grasps the Token in his pocket and takes a couple of deep, centering breaths. A new strength courses through him, and he lets go of the railing.

Bridge Body-Mind Connecting Features

The Bridge has built-in design features for catalyzing the threshold experience. Employing the body-mind connection, these features create physical responses that open pathways for parallel responses in the mind. Here is each design feature and what it can potentially cause:

- ▶ **Abrupt Changes of Direction before the Bridge.** Activates new neural pathways, which creates an opening for new possibilities.

- ▶ **The Bridge Itself.** As a transition zone between two landmasses, it instills a level of uncertainty and begs curiosity.

- ▶ **Wooden Plank Walkway.** A level of trust is needed for stepping out into thin air, supported only by a slat of wood.

- ▶ **Steep Entry Incline.** Along with activating new neural pathways, looking upward and the extra exertion hint at the effort needed for this quest.

- ▶ **Railing.** The dance between self-reliance and support—and the sense of safety—are each going to play roles.

- ▶ **Level Center, Suspended over Water.** A glance downward says that the feeling of relaxation at the apex of the arch is tenuous. A Journey is movement, and movement means risk and change.

- ▶ **Panoramic View between Two Worlds.** The vista instills a sense of comfort and spaciousness, which relaxes and opens the mind.

- ▶ **Steep Exit Decline.** More neural pathways not regularly used come into play, along with the sense of descending into something new.

THE SHADOW SIDE OF THINGS

On first impression, the Bridge spans a wetland. Yet it is much wetter than appearance would have it. The vegetation forms a floating mat, which masks two to three feet of water underneath. Here is the first of Nature's many trailside lessons that things aren't always as they appear.

As Chris steps off the Bridge and onto the Trail, he has to turn either right or left. Tacked to a post in front of him is a rustic arrow made of White Birch sticks. It points to the left. He realizes he'd have gone that way anyway, because it will take him around the Trail in a clockwise direction. That, according to the *Forest Bathing Companion* book, will heighten his sensory awareness and magnify Nature's healing energies, because he will be flowing in harmony with them.

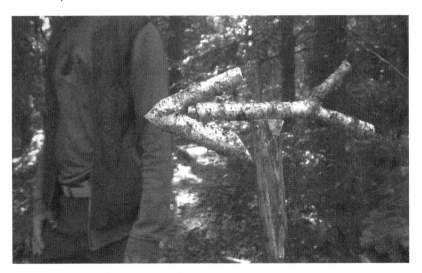

The only Trail sign

The regional Ojibwe call doing things in a clockwise fashion Walking the Sun Trail. Both Sun and Moon travel clockwise (which they call "sunwise") across the sky. They say the Path of Life follows the Sun Trail by starting at birth in the East, the direction of new beginnings, then ending in the West, where we ultimately go to join the Ancestors when we pass over from this life. The Ojibwe and many other indigenous people enter ceremonial circles—and conduct their lives in general—in a sunwise fashion.

Chris takes his first tentative steps on the Trail, feeling uplifted by the thought that he could be following the tradition of his Ancestors and others who live in balance with Earth's energies.

CHAPTER FIVE

Sensitizing with Breath

I inhale, she exhales

She exhales, I inhale

She breathes into me,

I breathe into her

Her breath is my life,

My breath is her life

We need each other,

The Tree and me

We are one breath,

We are one body

Chris crosses the little bridge over the Beaver Canal and immediately the Trail takes him atop a knoll crowned with Elder Pines. The view of the dappled forest floor rolling down the knoll to the south and the Blue Iris-bejeweled bog to the north takes his breath away, then tempts him to take in one of theirs.

"Drink it all in," whispers Chris's Guide, Sarah, not wanting to break the spell. The two of them had agreed to meet up on Breathing Knoll, and he's glad she's there to share the moment with him.

The way she just gently interjected reminds Chris that when he first met her, she told him that her primary role would be to help him personalize his relationship with Nature. Beyond that, she said she'd remain as transparent as possible; she wouldn't get in the way.

The Original Aromatherapy

"Take a few more breaths," she suggests. "Go slow and deep, all the way down into your gut and up into your sinuses.

"Now, breathe your next breath down through your pelvis, down your legs and into your feet. Feel it flowing through the soles of your feet and into the ground. You are now Rooted (see *Rooting* in chapter 8), and you can take in the nourishment of the Earth, just like the trees. And you can stand strong in a storm, just like the trees.

"And like the trees, you can exhale into the sky. Start deep in your gut, bringing up all that stale air, those toxic memories, and those hurtful behaviors. Bring them up through your chest, your throat, and out the top of your head. Let the cleansing breeze blow them away!"

After a few more cleansing breaths, Sarah asks Chris what he smells. He describes the piney essence given off by the surrounding trees basking in the midday sun. Every now and then, He catches a whiff of the cool, moss-freshened air wafting up from the bog below. He takes another deep, conscious breath, and a smile spreads across his face as he basks in olfactory bliss.

"This is the original Aromatherapy," whispers Sarah. "Nature's special blend. Aromatherapy overlays the whole Trail experience. Here, breathing is healing—the air is dripping with body-mind medicine! Whether you're conscious of that or not, healing happens."

The Timeless Breath

Sarah motions for Chris to come over and sit with her under the great Red Pine (*Pinus resinosa*) that towers above everything else atop the knoll. Even if his eyes were closed, he's sure he could still feel the pine's stately presence.

"We're here to become fluent in silence," Sarah softly states. "There is a language that the trees and the animals and the Earth speak, that we hear when we listen with our nose and eyes and ancestral mind. We call it Naturespeak. Linear time disappears. Objects take on new forms." (For more on Naturespeak, see *Becoming Nature: Learning the Language of Wild Animals and Plants,* by Tamarack Song).

"We can then see this great tree as the Earth breathing. The tree reaches up and expands as the Earth inhales, then contracts back to the soil as She exhales. One breath can take hundreds of years, so recognizing it as a breath falls beyond our normal grasp. On this Walk, let us listen with our whole beings, and we will begin to hear the whole story of life."

Chris stares in awe, realizing that he will never look at a tree—or perhaps anything else—in the same way again. The awareness makes him wonder what this could mean for his healing.

After a moment, Sarah continues, "If you can embrace this perspective right off the bat, it could change your entire Trail experience. We typically see things not as they are, but as we are. With a Naturespeak mindset, we can see not only new possibilities, but a new world. We'll come to realize that our old world was largely a construct of our conditioning that disguised so much of what we could have been seeing and experiencing."

Breathing in Earth and Trees

After another respectful moment's pause, Sarah motions Chris to part the pine needle carpet and scoop up a small handful of the dark, moist earth beneath. Following her example, he holds it to his nose, breathing moist, warm air into it. Inhaling the musty-yet-sweet fragrance the soil gives back, he repeats it several times, wanting to make sure he carries the aroma-memory with him.

The two of them circle around to the sunny side of the trunk, where she has him breathe into the bark while cupping his hands around his nose. "That's so you can capture and inhale what the tree gives back," she says. "Its healing balm is like no other—it enriches body, mind, and spirit.

"When you need stronger support," Sarah adds, "pick a few needles and crush them between your palms. Then take in the essence with a slow, full, deep-belly breath, always through the nose."

> **If you have allergies or a sinus condition** and struggle to breathe through your nose, take a decongestant or neti pot sinus rinse before your Walk. If that does not help, you can still benefit from Aromatherapy, though at a slower rate than if you could breathe normally.

Conscious Breathing Intentions

"Let's take what we've opened up to here along with us," says Sarah as the two of them get up to continue on the Trail. "But before we go, I invite you to breathe along with me and energize our intentions ...

Breathe in awareness; breathe out numbness.
Breathe in initiative; breathe out indifference.
Breathe in joy; breathe out despair.
Breathe in healing essences; breathe out toxins.
Breathe in nurturing relationships; breathe out exploitation.
Breathe in Nature; breathe out separation.
Breathe in love; breathe out love."

Tree Canopy Aromatherapy

As Chris moves on, Sarah tells him about an adaptation of a traditional healing-breath practice that is available at select Healing Nature Trails, including this one. A licensed Recreational Rope

Tree Climbing Instructor takes him up into the treetops, where the trees' healing essences are particularly potent.

"It's called *Tree Canopy Aromatherapy*," Sarah says, "and you don't have to have prior training in order to do it. However, it does take scheduling well in advance, and it is weather dependent."

Chris's heart skips a beat as you imagine being cradled high in the upper branches of an immense Elder Pine. *What must it be like*, he wonders, *to be in the treetops with the Birds, gently swaying in the breeze as you become intoxicated with essences coming straight off of the boughs all around you?*

Reading his feelings, Sarah asks Chris if he ever climbed trees as a child.

He nods.

"This isn't a whole lot different, except that you do it with ropes, harnesses, helmets, and pulleys," explains Sarah. "The focus is on safety, for both the climber and the trees.

"Once you're harnessed and clipped on your rope, you can ascend at your own pace, and you're able to move around the tree more than you might imagine. You might want to just sit and enjoy the view, or you can swing, stand on a limb, or go up into the canopy.

"Whatever you choose to do, the moment your feet leave the ground, you are moving in a new, exhilarating way that creates new, exhilarating possibilities for your inner processes. It's a phenomenal way to take advantage of the body-mind connection.

"Even with that, most people say that watching a tree rock back and forth in the breeze is one thing, but rocking with it is an other-worldly experience!"

Walking the Medicine Stick

"You may not be floating in the treetops this time," says Sarah, "yet you can take some of that energy with you on your Walk. These sticks here on the ground hold the memories of many dances in the sunshine, and of being whipped around by many a violent storm. Their buds have held the promise of new life through cold, cold winters, and their lush leaves have nurtured Caterpillars and shaded nestling Birds.

"In the autumn, they released their leaves to the forest floor, knowing the protective carpet was needed to protect their Forest kin who slept beneath until spring. The twigs stood bare to the Arctic blasts and bitter-cold nights, trusting that warm breezes and sweet sap would again come to swell their buds and renew the Dance of Life.

"There is an ancient healing tradition called *Walking the Medicine Stick*. Lying under an Elder Tree you find a dead stick—one who wishes to guide you with her stories of what she's seen and done; One who is weathered and porous enough to absorb your pain and take on the memories you wish to release. You Walk your Healing Trail carrying the stick in your left hand, which is your giving hand as it is the one closest to your heart.

"As you Walk, you might feel your tortured history, with all its misery, flowing out of your body and into the stick. And even if you don't feel it, it still happens. The stick is glad and honored to serve in this way, as it is her purpose to take the stories of the storms and the Caterpillars and the nestlings—and your stories—back to Mother Earth to be composted. Once they are broken down, their elements will be taken up as nourishment to support new life and new stories, based on the strength and wisdom of the old.

"The traditional ritual way to be involved in the process is to break the stick in half at the end of your Walk, then reverently lay the stick in the Fire. The breaking and burning is an act of empowerment that releases you from the clutches of victimization. You are then free to walk on—cleansed, refreshed, and rebirthed into your new life."

Chris has no question on what to do—a Medicine Stick whose furrowed surface says she has seen many turns of the seasons atop the tree calls out to him, and he firmly grasps her in his left hand.

The Trail's Healing Breath

Chris reads in *The Forest Bathing Companion* that he will have the opportunity to bathe in the healing breath of numerous aromatic herbs and trees. Already he spotted Monarda Mint (*Monarda fistulosa*), Evening Primrose (*Oenothera biennis*), and Sweet Fern (*Comptonia peregrina*) in the pollinator flowerbeds at the entrance, and in the Gateway Labyrinth Path dividers. Now that he's in the Forest, he comes across the red berries and shiny perennial leaves of Wintergreen (*Gaultheria procumbens*).

While Sarah describes the growth characteristics and healing properties of these herbs, she reminds Chris about the Elder Red Pine he met atop Breathing Knoll. "Look up," she says, "and see how many other kinds of trees you notice. Most of them have healing properties," she adds, "and we're benefiting from them right now. There's Yellow Birch (*Betula alleghaniensis*), White Pine (*Pinus strobus*), Tamarack (*Larix laricina*), Black Spruce (*Picea mariana*), and—as you can see all around us—the abundant Balsam Fir (*Abies balsamea*)."

Chris comments that the warm afternoon makes it all the easier for him to go barefoot. "That's good," says Sarah. "If you were wearing heavy footwear, it would insulate you from the full Grounding effect of the Earth's electromagnetic energy. Grounding can amplify the peaceful, euphoric feeling you are already experiencing from the pheromones given off by the trees. Adding to it are the negative ions being generated by the trees and flowing water. And let's not forget the added bonus: your immune system is being boosted."

"Now, if it was getting toward evening," Sarah continues, "or even if it was a cloudy day, we could stop to watch this Evening Primrose open her flowers in slow motion—a natural movie. The chemical compounds you would smell in the blossom were used by the local Ojibwe to help heal wounds and bruises. Today, the blossom extract is used to ease the symptoms of premenstrual syndrome.

"Over here are some Sweet Fern bushes. Go ahead and bruise a leaf, but be prepared to be inundated with a delightful, spicy aroma. It makes a great invigorating tea, which many people find to be delicious. Traditionally, Sweet Fern was used to line berry-gathering baskets, to repel bees and other insects that were attracted by the sweet berries.

"Then right at your feet you'll notice Wintergreen, which you may know. Most people know the refreshing essence—it's *methyl salicylate*, which has long been used to treat muscle pain. It's essentially the same compound found in aspirin.

"This Yellow Birch over here has similar properties. Just scratch a twig with your fingernail, and the tree will release a fragrance that is nearly identical to Wintergreen's. In days past, Yellow Birch was commonly tapped for her syrup, which was used for medicine, and as a flavoring.

"I bet you already know that the needles of most conifers are high in vitamin C. The White Pine, which you see towering above us here, was best known in the old days for keeping scurvy at bay. A vitamin C power tea is made from seeping the crushed needles in warm water.

Bad Breath for Biting Bugs

A few mosquitoes are buzzing around Chris's head, so he pulls out the natural insect repellent he brought along. Sarah takes note and says, "If you look at the ingredients, I bet you'll see that they come from plants like those we're getting to know here along the Trail. You might be surprised to hear that most of this vegetation produces insect-repelling substances. If you didn't bring any repellent with you, you could just go directly to the source. Nearly all strongly aromatic plant essences repulse insects. All you have to do is the same thing we did for Aromatherapy: crush the leaves or needles between the palms of your hands, only rub the oils you extracted directly on your skin, rather than inhaling them."

"What about the Balsam Fir?" Chris asks. "It sure would be handy if they worked, because they're everywhere."

"It's almost as though we saved the best for last," Sarah replies. "It's true; here in the Northcountry, it seems as though you're never more than a few steps away from a Fir tree. She has many secrets to share with us—secret to most of us, anyway. The Ojibwe rely heavily on this tree, whom they refer to as *Elder Sister*. Her sap, which is antibacterial and antiseptic, can be used to treat cuts, scrapes, and lesions. It's easy to obtain; just pop one of these resin-filled boils on the bark, which as you can see are numerous.

"The sap also makes a good cold and headache treatment. Put a dab on your upper lip, so that you can continually inhale the essence. The Ojibwe inhale the steam-extracted essence from the needles and many others treat colds with a tea made from either the needles or the sap."

"What about Balsam Fir's insect repellent properties?" Chris asks. "That's what I'm most interested in right now."

"I can understand why; I could use some of her help myself! Fortunately, there are several options to choose from to fit the situation. The volatile oils in the needles make a good insect repellent, which can be either rubbed directly on the skin from the crushed needles, or you can use the essential oil that is available for purchase. If mosquitoes are biting through your hair and clothing, you can let them absorb the heavy smoke produced from placing the boughs on a smoldering fire. Or, for a fragrantly fashionable look, tuck a few fresh boughs under your hat brim, so that they drape loosely over your face."

Sarah chooses the last option. Chris follows her lead, and he's surprised at how well it works.

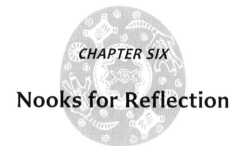

CHAPTER SIX

Nooks for Reflection

"**B**y the way," says Sarah, "take note of any special places along the Trail where you feel naturally relaxed, and that appeal to your sense of aesthetic. It might be where we sat on the soft needles under that great Pine, or out on one of the points that have beautiful overviews. Or it could be a quiet nook. Some people find a *Power Spot*—a place with healing or revitalizing energy. Some others find a place that they think sits on a *Ley Line*, which is an alignment of landforms or places of spiritual significance. It just has to be a place that speaks especially to you."

Comfort Spots

"We generally refer to these special places as *Comfort Spots*. For many who've been here on the Trail, their Comfort Spots have become valuable partners in their healing processes."

"How so?" Chris asks.

"For some, it's a familiar place to return to, where they know they can find the solace or inspiration they need. Yet for many others, they don't have to be physically present to benefit. Imagine you're meditating and you want to visualize a peaceful place to help bring you to a state of mindfulness; your Comfort Spot could do the trick."

"Are there any ways to use a Comfort Spot remotely for healing?"

"You bet! I have a client who envisions being at her Comfort Spot when she gets stressed at work. It calms her right down, she says. And Comfort Spots can be a big help for people working through trauma. When trauma memories surface, they close their eyes and go to their Comfort Spots. Over time, this helps them let go of their stories, as their special place on the Mother's bosom helps them to realize that it's possible to feel safe and supported."

"It sounds like these people are creating a Comfort Spot within," Chris muses. What a beautiful way to return to Nature, by having Nature return to you!"

To Visualize Your Comfort Spot Remotely

Close your eyes and take several deep, slow breaths. If you can, either go outside away from traffic, or listen to a recording of Nature sounds. Let the images and sensations of your Comfort Spot drift into your consciousness. Look around and notice particular objects, such as a fallen log or patch of blueberries. Smell the pregnant air and feel the soft breeze in your face. Stay there until your heart is calmed. For more on this technique, see Remote Walking in chapter 14.

Regarding the Beaver Tree

On the north side of the island, the Trail dips low and skirts the Spruce bog. Sarah stops and, pointing with her gaze, has Chris looking inland from the bog toward a large dead tree. He wonders why she died, as other than having no leaves, she looks to be in her prime.

Then he notices it; a little over a foot off the ground, her trunk is girdled about two-thirds of the way through. Chris is surprised she's still standing.

"Who did this?" Chris asks.

"Beaver," Sarah responds.

"How do you know that?"

"We Trail Guides all have naturalist training so we can use Examples from Nature as metaphors."

"Neat. So maybe you know the answer to my next question: Why didn't they finish the job?"

"Do you have any unfinished business in your life?"

That hit Chris right between the eyes. He realizes that it's so easy for him to see other people's inadequacies and failings. And it's so easy to make excuses for his own.

"Let's sit down here for a while," Chris tells Sarah. "I've got some work to do."

"Before you start," replies Sarah, "see that Hemlock sapling over there that's a little shorter than you? How old do you think she is?"

"I would guess eight or ten years. But the way you asked the question, I'm prepared to be surprised—like with the invisible three-foot deep water under the Threshold Bridge."

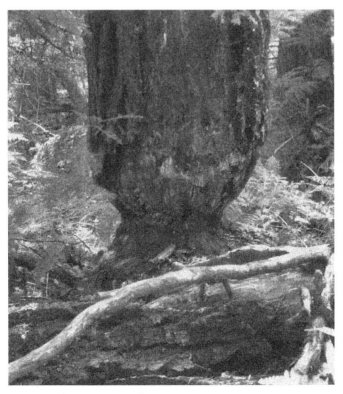

The Beaver Tree metaphor

"You're right. Here's another example of things not only in Nature, but in life, being more—or other—than they initially appear. That little Hemlock, that's no more than the diameter of your little finger, is probably 100 years old. If she were growing in the open, she'd be so big that you couldn't get your arms around her. Instead, she's biding her time while she grows in wisdom and resilience. Then, when an overhead tree topples and creates an opening, she'll have the wherewithal to shoot up into the light."

"Now that's a potent metaphor! Unfinished business …failings … inadequacies … I wonder what's under them …"

A Trail Divided

After Chris processes the metaphor of the Tree, he feels as though he's done a day's work. Yet he knows he's just begun—that the Beaver Tree just gave him a doorway to the real work. Without being called on how he became blinded to himself by projecting on others, he knows from past counseling work that he would just be going through the motions if he continued on the Trail. He reminds himself that the first step on any Healing Journey has to be taking personal responsibility for his state of being.

Right away this realization is put to the test, as the Trail forks. Sarah stands back as Chris ponders. He doesn't want to risk getting lost or missing anything, so he consults the map. It shows the left-hand fork, which is the main Trail, going straight ahead and taking him to Trail features he read about—features that he looks forward to taking advantage of.

The map, however, just shows the beginning of the right-hand fork—the Discovery Fork. How long it is, where it will ultimately take him, and what he might or might not experience, are all a mystery.

"I get it," Chris tells himself. "Sometimes the straight and narrow, the known entity, is the way to go. However, that's not why I came. Familiarity may bring comfort, but not anymore—not for me. The same old, same old, has grown thin."

A Joseph Campbell line enters Chris's mind: "We must be willing to get rid of the life we've planned, so as to have the life that is waiting for us." Chris came here to step into the Void: that place where all that he knows dissolves into a formless, shapeless mélange. He wants to strip down to the essence and question everything. It's no longer good enough to just get by; he wants what works.

Yet there is apprehension. It brings up another line from Joseph Campbell: "The cave you fear to enter holds the treasure you seek." The treasure ...that's it! As Campbell would put it, Chris wants to follow his bliss—he wants to feel his feet solidly under him and his heart dancing for the sheer joy of being alive!

He takes the Discovery Fork.

The Havens

When the Discovery Fork brings Chris back to the main Trail, Sarah tells him that the Trail has its shadow side. "While it facilitates movement and direction," she says, "the Trailside Havens offer places to withdraw and slow down. While the Trail is a venue for external exploration, the Havens foster the Inner Journey. 'Here in solitude and peace my soul was nurst, amid the loveliest scenes of unpolluted nature,' said Robert Southey, who was a 19th-century poet laureate of England. Rather than being the movement, you have the opportunity in the Havens to reflect on the movement within and around you."

Sarah goes on to say that all five Havens offer beautiful settings, Grounding benches, and gated privacy. The gates are unobtrusive—they're just dead branches placed across the entryway Paths. Four of the Havens open to panoramic vistas. Experiencing the expansiveness of the view plies upon the body-mind connection, which helps open mind and heart to new possibilities. One of those possibilities is the avenue provided for the release of pent-up stress and emotional baggage.

"Yet it's not just a vista," says Sarah, "it's the sense of awe that comes with it. The view alone doesn't work—especially if you see it regularly. You have to be drawn into it and swept away by it."

"What if I'm just too self-absorbed or numbed-out to get into it?"

"What can help is a dynamic meditation called *Coming to Oneness* that Tamarack the Trail's co-founder, Tamarack Song, learned from the Seneca people. It instills that sense of awe by taking you out of yourself—beyond your ego—and projecting you into the Circle of Life. It's also a good stress release, and a way to relax around troubles and open to new possibilities. Coming to Oneness works particularly well with panoramic vistas because they're a part of the meditation. Together they instill a sense of awe that becomes transcendent."

"Hmm ...Can you teach it to me?"

"Sure—it's easy. All you do is focus on something small that catches your attention, like that Caterpillar there. Before long, you notice the Oxeye Daisy she's perched on, then the whole bed of Daisies. Now you see that Butterfly visiting the flowers, and the Bees. Look at that Bee taking off, maybe for the flowers over on the rise to the south. Now I see you're looking east, at the three Swans who just landed on the Beaver pond. See how, before you know it, you get taken in by the wonder of it all? By consciously narrowing your focus, you created the dynamic tension to expand into the Oneness."

"You're right, it's easy—it just happens. Thanks for that. But it seems to be the opposite of meditation: instead of turning inward, you expand outward."

"From Zen perspective," replies Sarah, "the distinction between the two is only a construct of the mind. When we use one as an avenue to the other, we reunite them into their original oneness."

Going back to describing the Havens, Sarah says they are typically used for:

❱ Reflection and Sitting Meditation.

❱ Therapist-client work.

❱ Lunch and a short rest.

❱ Half-day or day-long retreats.

She goes on to say that each Haven has its distinctive features, which contribute to the unique experience it has to offer:

1. **Red Pine Refuge.** Tucked into the deep forest behind the Breathing Knoll, this special place features two benches nestled between Elder Pines.

2. **Frog Pond Point.** Being right down at bog level, Chris can commune with this most unique and mysterious of Northwoods habitats by being able to see, smell, and touch it.

3. **Stump Labyrinth Outlook.** Perched atop the base of a fallen tree is a Finger Labyrinth weathered by the seasons and the touch of many hands. The healing energy is strong here, with much support from the Otters, Swans, and other wildlings in the waters that lap the point.

4. **Beaver Dam Waters.** Tumbling over the dam from the Beaver Pond into the channels of the Aquarinth below, water healing energy is strong here. Chris can sit next to the spillway and bathe in negative ions, or immerse himself in the pond for Water Grounding (see chapter 8).

5. **Solitude Sundeck.** On a quiet peninsula between the Aquarinth and Zen Untangle is a private pier with a mosquito net canopy. It is ideal for therapeutic sunbathing, meditation, and reflective reading; and it is a favorite place for therapists to bring their clients.

Frog Pond, Red Pine, and Solitude Sundeck can be reserved for therapist sessions and retreats.

Since it's Chris's first time on the Trail, he tells Sarah that he wants to see and experience all the Havens. She understands his curiosity and enthusiasm, and at the same time she reminds him that he is here for a reason. "Getting to know all five of the Havens could take a day in itself," she says. "I suggest you choose one now that you think would best serve your work. Then after your Walk, you might have time to get to know some of the others."

Gathering at the Pine Grove Circle

Just before the canoe livery for the Aquarinth, Chris notices a side Trail leading into a Virgin Pine Grove. He is entranced—he can't help but follow his impulse.

It turns out to be a very short Trail, ending in a circle of log benches. *What an idyllic place for small-group meetings*, he muses as his bare feet sink into the thick carpet of golden pine needles.

Then he looks up.

His eyes follow the bark's craggy creases upward, upward, upward, until his gaze gets lost in far-above ferny branchlets wafting in the breeze. The only sky he sees is what manages to peek through spaces in the ever-moving canopy. The scene is framed by a circle of russet columns that must be what the creators of Stonehenge were trying to equal. It steals his breath.

He feels dizzy and lightheaded, and he has to sit down. "You can see why this is a popular destination," says Sarah after allowing him a short while to soak in the ambience. "Sometimes a few Trail Walkers will get together here and share with each other what they are experiencing. More often than not, they learn from each other's experiences. And they inspire and support each other.

"But the main users of this Circle are healthcare practitioners with their groups, workshop presenters, and spiritual communities. Families also like coming here to reconnect or work on issues with their therapists. Yet whoever it is and whatever their purpose, nearly everyone comes because they find that the steadfast and wisdom-rooted Elder Energy does wonders in facilitating their process."

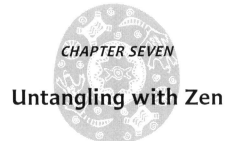

CHAPTER SEVEN

Untangling with Zen

"We're now two-thirds of the way through our Journey," announces Sarah as the two step back on the main Trail. "I see you're still struggling for a breakthrough. I wonder if you might be trying too hard. Listening takes relaxing, and making sense of new information often takes new pathways to process it. The ancient sages of the Far East knew this and came up with the method of inquiry through non-inquiry that cuts to the quick."

"Tell me more," Chris says. "I meditate and I've been a casual student of Zen, but I have a hunch that, from what I've seen so far, the folks who designed this Trail have come up with a unique way to use Zen to crack open Nature."

"There's no reason to come up with anything," Sarah replies, "because Nature is already Zen—essential Zen, that is—before Zen took on characteristics of the established spiritual practices of the time."

She goes on to explain the way of essential Zen, which is "to release yourself to the Void: the realm that is neither within nor without, neither above nor below. There is no form or shape, no light nor dark, and nothing to hang onto. To Enter the Void is to freefall, with no expectations and no safety net. Nothing matters: belief, desire—even strength of will—can gain no foothold. There is no past or future, and everything that anchors you in the present has been rendered null and … void.

"With the final three Labyrinthine Experiences: the Aquarinth, the Zen Untangle, and the Zen Garden, which we collectively refer to as the *Zen Trilogy*, there is no set form or shape. They take you into the Void, where anything is possible. You are no longer bound by your past, nor are you enslaved to your future. True change is now possible, and these three Labyrinths can help you craft it."

Experience 1: Paddling the Meanders of the Aquarinth

Almost immediately, Chris comes upon a thatch-roofed gazebo off to the side of the Trail. It reminds him of something he'd see in a tropical Native village. Inside are four canoes: two solo boats, a small tandem, and a wooden dugout, which he can't take his eyes off of.

Sarah notices. "It was hewn out of the trunk of an old, old White Pine who was laid down by a storm. The paddle was carved from the same tree. A member of our staff, crafted them—they're replicas of what the Natives here used to make."

"With the heritage behind that boat," muses Chris, "she has to have stories to tell, especially with how ancient the tree must've been that she came from."

"Yeah, people who've been out on the water with her say she has quite the wisdom to share."

On the opposite side of the Trail is a canoe launch. Chris has been waiting for this, as he is a water person, and he was hoping that some connection with water will help him make a breakthrough.

"First, some background," says Sarah. "Awareness is the first step in healing; it's what makes it possible for us to be consciously engaged in the process. Water, as I'm sure you know, is the universal solvent. It likes to absorb and diffuse whatever comes its way. Variable in its form, water seeks a common level, and it adapts easily to new surroundings. And it changes easily to fit its surroundings. All things immersed in water are equally embraced, and all things floating upon its surface are equally supported. Could there be any better metaphor for the Healing Journey?

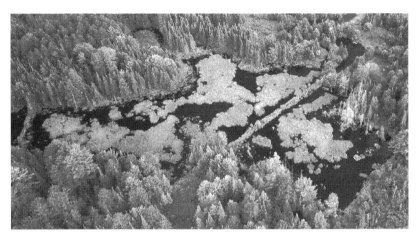

The Aquarinth

"When we submerge in water, glide over it, or merely dangle our feet in it, we intuitively know that we are being unconditionally accepted. There is no judgment or expectation; we are embraced and cherished for just who and how we are. She is there for us, giving a format for our quest, amplifying our every effort, and clarifying the voices we hear."

Sarah goes on to tell Chris that the canoe launch takes him directly out to the Aquarinth, which is comprised of a network of meandering waterways that fork, rejoin, and dead-end. The waterscape is sprinkled with floating islands of sedges, lilies, and cranberries.

"Our Aquarinth may be the only one in the state," she says, "and perhaps the country. We couldn't find another one anywhere."

Back to the description, Sarah tells Chris that the way of the Aquarinth is a slow and sinuous paddle around the murky backwaters of the mind. There is no marked route, and there is no center to reach, as with the Gateway Labyrinth. Instead, this one is for listening. There is nothing to fix, nothing to heal, and nowhere in particular to go. The experience is completely open to where he needs to go in order to find those lost parts of himself.

This unique experience is best suited for people like Chris, continues Sarah, who are ready to relax their boundaries and to listen to the quiet murmurings of their souls. The expansiveness of the wetland, the quiet depths of the waters, the free flight of the birds, and the wind singing in the shoreline trees all encourage openness, inquisitiveness, and a sense of reverence.

"Yet not everybody is a water person," Sarah explains. "And some need perspective more than introspection. For them, you'll see up in that tree the equivalent of the Cosmorinth, only this one overlooks the Aquarinth. We call it the Osprey Nest."

She points to a ladder leading up to a small observation deck. Chris can't resist; he climbs up to get a view, which makes him feel like he could spread his wings and rise above the tangle in which he finds himself.

Yet he knows escape is not what he's here for—he must go down and immerse himself in the riverine mind-maze. The boat slips quietly into the water, and he lets it take him wherever he need to go.

Experience 2: Breaking Through in the Zen Untangle

Chris's time on the water leaves him feeling more comfortable in his own skin than he's been in a long time. But it's not enough. Shaming voices keep spinning around in his consciousness. *You should be at work. Why didn't you finish your degree? Why did you keep that secret?* Chris tells Sarah what's haunting him, and that he's ready to give up.

Her body language says to follow her. They pass the turnoff to the Solitude Sundeck and soon come to another side Path. Sarah steps aside and motions for him to go first.

The Path ascends several feet to a flat-topped rise that is about thirty feet in diameter and neatly bordered with birch logs. In its center stands a middle-aged White Pine. The ground around it is strewn with an array of boulders, driftwood, and tree stumps.

"This is what my head feels like," Chris tells Sarah.

"You're not the first one who sees this as a metaphor for their knotted-up mind and bottled-up emotions. When people come

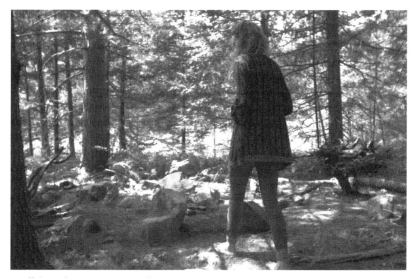

Walking the Zen Untangle

here to the Trail to reach a state of deep and undefended consciousness, and they haven't achieved it by this point, they're often ready to pack out, just like you. Some of them lament about how they're still stuck in old thought patterns, or how they're unable to break through self-imposed psycho-emotional boundaries. This place, the Zen Untangle, is able to help most of them break through. It's got such a reputation that some folks come just for the Untangle. Some people find it so helpful for clearing their minds that they return on a regular basis. For them, it's a pilgrimage. We have a few who come weekly."

How It Works

"But why?" Chris asks. "What makes this experience so special?"

"Some folks feel a concentration of energy here," Sarah replies. "They call it a Power Spot or a confluence of Ley Lines, similar to some people's Comfort Spots, which we talked about a little further back on the Trail. The founders of the Trail first saw something special in this site because they were drawn by all the animal signs. They found an observation platform about twenty feet up in this Pine in the middle of the Untangle, which showed that a previous owner must also have been drawn to this spot. And the founders noticed that the Path leading up to the rise came from the north, which in Ojibwe tradition is the direction of introspection and guidance."

"That all sounds great," Chris replies, "but I still don't get how this tangle of sticks and stones is going to help me untangle."

"I'm not surprised. Again, it's all about the body-mind connection, which as you now know is so strong that the body's movements and rhythms are mirrored in the mind, and vice versa. This makes it possible to use the body as a doorway to the mind. So when we are muddled in confusion, we can use physical movement to help unravel the tangle.

"It's done by meandering around and between the boulders and stumps in random fashion. Avoid stepping in the same place twice, and continually look for new Pathways. Once you get the hang of it, quit thinking about where you shouldn't go and just allow yourself to move free-form, without rhyme or reason.

"In essence, what makes the exercise work is that we are using random movement to relax the mental patterns that keep us trapped in the same thought and feeling loops. This allows for greater emotional expression and the ability to visualize new possibilities. Repressed feelings and forgotten memories often surface. The avoidance patterns and boundaries that keep us from being fully conscious begin to dissolve. Along with that, sensory acuity and mental sharpness increase."

Sarah stresses the fact that that the key is *aimless meandering*, which means *with no pattern and no goal in mind*. "Goal orientation keeps us emotionally numb and married to our past," she says. "Fortunately, this unique Labyrinth makes aimlessness pretty easy to achieve. With the stumps and boulders placed in no particular order, you'd have to try hard to go the same way twice in a row."

Why It Works

Chris asks Sarah how much time she recommends that he meander around in the Untangle in order to get his mind untangled.

"To have my answer make sense, let me first explain the science behind it. Let's start with the relationship between short-term and long-term memory. What we think and perceive is first held in our short-term memory. In order for it to be converted to long-term memory, it has to have either made a lasting impression on us, or we have to give it attention. That has to happen within fifteen minutes; otherwise, it gets swept away, and it's gone forever.

"By having to be constantly engaged in where you place your next step, lest you stumble and fall on a rock, it's impossible to keep focused on those same old crippling thoughts and draining feelings that have been haunting you. So after fifteen minutes, your short-term memory is filled with only vague impressions of countless random movements.

"The neural synapses that govern your patterned psycho-emotional responses—that nagging mental clutter—have now had time to relax. This allows for a broader range of thought and feeling than you've been experiencing. There is space for repressed memories to surface and for old stories to be given a new interpretation.

"And what some folks, including therapists, find most liberating is the opportunity to escape entrenched thought-conclusion loops, which means that one continues to use a thought or memory to verify the reality it reflects. Some therapists bring their clients here for that breakthrough experience alone.

"Another important factor is that it can take some time for the body-mind connection to fully activate. For many people, it takes only a few minutes. Yet there are some so wounded and defensive that they need to spend two or three days here on the Trail before they start breaking through. The Zen Untangle speeds up the process for nearly everybody.

"Even those who are doing well by the time they get to this point on the Trail enjoy the Untangle because they say it helps them feel even freer, and more relaxed and engaged, than they already were. For some people, the Untangle turns out to be a threshold experience; having gained perspective and realizing things that previously escaped them, they go on with new hope."

Freshly Untangled

Sarah waits for Chris back where the Untangle Path meets the main Trail. "I can tell by your serene look that the magic worked," she says. His soft smile is all she needs for confirmation.

"One reason you feel the way you do," she adds, "is that you're leaving the Untangle through the Northern Gateway, which from native perspective empowers the Inner Journey and brings new awarenesses. This is possible because, in contemporary terms, you have re-centered by shifting from your rational mind-based memory to your limbic mind, which is the home of your intuition, emotions, and deep-seated memories.

"Now, with a fresh slate and limbered-up mental processes, you may finally be ready for Nature's guidance and healing embrace. At this point, I sometimes suggest that people go back to the Trail entrance sign and start over. It's often those who are struggling with addiction or have been trapped in extremely codependent relationships. Occasionally someone was blocked just because she wasn't accustomed to being deep in Nature. However, I think you can continue from here, as you've been able to engage yourself pretty well up to this point.

"Remember, though, that this is still a new beginning for you," Sarah cautions as Chris starts Walking. "New awareness is just hot air if it can't be acted upon. Just remember that every step is a new step—a fresh start."

Here again Chris sees that the Trail is designed to facilitate what is needed and when it is needed. Right away he finds himself crossing another one of the Trail's bridges, which supports leaving those old and all-too-familiar behavioral patterns behind. Passing over a bridge can also mean not getting mired in something that's best left behind, and moving on in new directions, to new heights.

"In fact, a fresh start is inevitable," says Sarah. "You'll see that the next few steps after the bridge take you up a short incline and right into a T-intersection. For the first time, you can't just lumber forward on the Trail. You have to choose going either left, to stay on the main Trail, or right, to take the Discovery Fork."

Chris recalls the words of philanthropist Margaret Shepard, "Sometimes the only available transportation is a leap of faith." He decides to stay on the main Trail. He now has clarity, and has his bearings, and he wants to stick with them.

Experience 3: Tending a Zen Garden

A tight curve takes Chris through a grove of small-diameter stumps, which are all that remain of saplings harvested by the resident Beaver colony. The coarse chew marks and decomposing condition of the stumps reminds him of what has come and gone in his life, yet rough-edged childhood trauma memories persist. Like those fading reminders of what could have been, Chris wants those old regrets and dashed dreams to transform into something fresh and fertile as well. He whispers a few words of gratitude for the breath of hope.

Again there is a quick change of direction in the Trail, followed immediately by a short section of Trail that hugs a slope. Chris thought he was quite present since leaving the Untangle, so he's surprised that he has to re-center himself and watch his step in order to keep from sliding off the Trail. Even so, he is thankful for this visceral reminder to not revert to his accustomed pattern of unconsciously plodding along in his mind.

"You might want to slow up here," says Sarah. "Out on the tip of this little peninsula on our left is a form of garden from the Far

East that is commonly known as a *Zen Garden*. If you're not familiar with the term, Zen Gardens are also known as *Dry Landscape Gardens, Japanese Rock or Sand Gardens, Contemplation Gardens,* and *Restorative Gardens.*

"The Zen Garden here is the wrap-up of the Zen Trilogy. It is the seventh and final Trail Labyrinth. It's another progression in the Labyrinthine Experience, which some people see as its ultimate expression."

Chris tells her that he's seen pictures of Zen Gardens, and maybe one in a movie, but never one in real life.

"They have quite the history," she continues. "Classical Shinto, Hindu, Daoist, and Buddhist traditions are represented here, among others. This type of Labyrinth evolved as a site for reflection and inspiration, and as a place to go on retreat. On occasion, a Zen Garden has served as a sanctuary.

"Think of such a Garden as a piece of Nature that has been isolated *from* Nature, yet it is still embraced *by* Nature. I know that sounds paradoxical, especially when you can see that this little Garden in front of us sits on a lush peninsula surrounded by a vibrant marsh, which is bordered by a dense conifer forest.

"Yet isn't that the paradox that many of us live? Even though our urbanized existence seems so differentiated from the rhythms and beauties of Nature, she is still our ultimate mother. And in essence we are nothing *but* Nature—and nothing *without* Nature.

"The Garden, then, meets us where we're at: we are children who've gotten lost, even though our mother was there all the time."

The Unpacking

"What you say resonates strongly with me," Chris replies. "I'd like to spend some time here—I think I need it. But first I really need some clarity. This looks more like a wannabe Garden to me; all I see is a glorified sandbox with a couple of garden tools and a pile of sticks and stones. How is this stuff going to help me reconnect?"

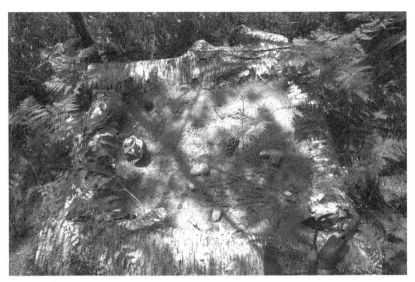

The Zen Garden

"You're right; this is a wannabe Garden. And you're at a gotta-do point in your life. The idea here is to bring wannabe and gotta-do together in order to bridge the gap between you and Nature. Which isn't so hard, really, because you already *are* Nature."

"Wow, I get it!" Chris exclaims. "My essential self is in attunement with Nature because it *is* Nature. I'm here to bring my conscious self into attunement with my essential self."

"That's a good way to put it," says Sarah. "Yet there's more to this sandbox. There's a German term, 'Auspacken,' that means to 'unpack,' as in emptying your suitcase. It also has a slang definition: to *unpack what's bothering you or what you're hiding*. When we say, 'Speak your mind!' or 'Come clean!' a German speaker might say, 'Auspacken!'

"I'm afraid you're losing me. I don't see why a Zen Garden is needed for that."

"The beauty of the Garden is that the unpacking is nonverbal. Sometimes people can't admit things to themselves, much less to others. Or they don't have words for it. Here is a way to express it by creating a landscape. It's a lot like art therapy: you just give your thoughts and feelings free reign to create what's going on inside."

"Ah, here's the body-mind connection again!" Chris states.

"Exactly. You have a blank slate here for graphic expression. Once you get going, a synergy develops; you move some sand and it shuffles something around in your mind, which dislodges a feeling, which in turn gives you the impulse to grab that dark stone and place it over there to the right, and so on. What you're doing is working with the core expressive archetypes of space, form, and intention."

"Are you saying, then, that this piece of raw Earth is like an artist's canvas, and my paints are the pebbles, sticks, pinecones, leaves, bones, and whatever else is at hand, and the rake and trowel are my brushes?"

"You've got it. And your intention is to manifest the landscape of your mind. You'll see that a maze of sorts emerges, which gives pathways for the mind and heart to wander and explore."

"But what if I get artist's block, so to speak?"

"Usually all it takes is touching the sand to start bringing form to the story. Just remember that the story is already there. Some envision the story to start with, and some just let the process flow."

Etching a Trauma Story

"Now that you've grasped the concept," says Sarah, "I'd like to tell you how a Zen Garden can be used in trauma recovery. As you may know, some people remember their traumatization stories, and some don't. Those who do are sometimes either too ashamed or too afraid of a Trauma Memory Response (a traumatic reaction brought on by a trauma-related trigger) to retell their stories. Those who don't remember may have been very young when they were traumatized, or they blotted out the conscious memory as a survival strategy.

"Whatever the case, it's an important step in many people's Healing Journeys to be able to recall and acknowledge their stories. Here is where the magic and mystique of the Zen Garden comes in—especially for those so drained by their trauma that they can't shed another tear. Sometimes someone has retreated so far into herself that she can't take a full breath. Or a therapist may come with a client who has sunk into deep depression, or who is contemplating suicide. I often bring them directly here, because there's something about a Zen Garden that encourages Auspacken.

"If Auspacken is possible, it could give them enough wherewithal to begin letting go of their stories. For so many, that is the critical next step in getting on with their recovery.

"It doesn't seem to matter whether their stories are right at the tips of their tongues or deeply buried in their somatic memories. What does matter is the opportunity to give form to the wordless, or to that which is too frightful to verbalize."

"So how do they give form to something they can't recall?" Chris asks.

"It may just be intuitive impressions guiding their hands," Sarah replies. "I typically start with Conscious Breathing, to help them relax into themselves and gain a sense of place. Then I'll use Aromatherapy to enliven their senses and bring them fully into the now. I might have them take a handful of ground from the Garden, breathe into it, then inhale the fertile, musty essence that the soil exudes. Or I'll suggest that they pick a few needles from a nearby conifer and inhale the fragrance they exude. That tends to stimulate the body-mind connection, and the storyteller's hand then begins the silent process of speaking the unspeakable. Their story takes shape before them, in a way that is both safe and recognizable.

"I can't begin to tell you what it's like to witness the miracle of someone expelling the story that has been haunting him for so long. There it is, laid out before him—it's no longer trapped in his head; it's no longer wracking his body. Sometimes my tears of relief flow right along with his, and sometimes I can't help but join him in dancing ecstatically around the Garden!"

"It must be an immensely rewarding experience for you as a Guide," Chris comments. "Yet it seems as though there is still some unfinished business. There he is, just him and his story. Then what?"

Ritual Release

"Then comes the most empowering part," Sarah says. "He is standing literally at his story's graveside, and he might need some time for mourning. Even though that story has stalked him mercilessly, it has also—for better or worse—helped form his identity. Walking away from that story could leave a void in his life. It's one of the reasons people stay in abusive relationships. So to see himself through the pain and uprootedness of separation, he needs some time to reconnect with his reason for leaving the story, along with renewed the courage to do so.

"Once he's done that, he can Walk on. He knows that Mother Earth will then play another role in his healing, by eroding away the story he left behind. There's a high chance that this approach will work for him, because he is walking away from something tangible, rather than just trying to escape the memory.

"Or he can erase the story himself, by whooshing it away with a bucket of water or—even more engaging—obliterating it with his bare hands. This is the approach used by Navajo healers with their sand paintings. A healer creates a symbolic painting from colored sand, then helps his or her patient imbue the painting with the essence of the sickness. The painting is then wiped away, and the strength of the sickness with it.

"The therapists I guide often recommend this active ritual release for their clients, because (as with so much of Nature's healing way) the hands-on component energizes the ritual and makes it more effective by bringing the body-mind connection into play.

"Therapists also tend to suggest the story-destruction approach to those who have been extremely victimized by their traumas. For those who have been so overpowered, this could be the most significant level of control over their situations that they've had.

"That's pretty much the overview. Is there anything else I can do before I leave you with your story?"

"You've already given me far more than I could have imagined," Chris replies. "I have a lot to reflect on. Thank you for the time you took with me. Being here on this spot with you has made your words all the more meaningful than if I had just read them."

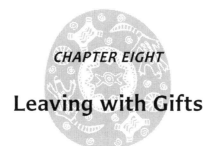

CHAPTER EIGHT

Leaving with Gifts

Chris returns to the Trail from the Zen Garden and immediately runs into a fork in the Trail. After the intensity of the Auspacken, he thought he'd be able to automatically relax into the comfort of the tried-and-true. But he sees that someone who had taken the Discovery Fork at the T-intersection just after the Zen Untangle rejoins the main Trail right where he is standing, only to face the same decision he now has before him.

It's not, however, the same type of decision as with past Discovery Forks. Here Chris can see some distance ahead on both Trails. The Main Trail would take him under the biggest White Pine he's ever seen, then across three short bridges that wrap around a marshy bay. The Discovery Fork, on the other hand, crosses a long, low bridge that cuts across to the far shore of the bay.

Something inside nags at Chris, and he feels on edge. He fully expected to be Walking on with a sense of accomplishment, but now he wrestles with some dark urge to reenter the Void and continue the open-discover-release process.

A Bridge over Troubled Water

As Chris approaches the long Bridge, he realizes why he felt edgy when he looked down upon it from the fork in the Trail: the Bridge has no railing.

But he can't blame his edginess on the Bridge. After all, one of the reasons he came here is to learn how to take more personal responsibility for his life, and externalizing on the Bridge would just feed his all-too-familiar feelings of helplessness.

"Ha! Here's the body-mind connection at work again," Chris says to himself. "The Trail designers probably placed this edgy-looking Bridge here right after the Zen Garden to keep people like me from sinking into complacency. It could well be that I have more work to do."

It doesn't take Chris more than a couple of steps on the Bridge to realize that it's not just edgy looking. It has a bounce to it that makes him feel insecure. "I'm sure it's safe," he tells himself, but he slows down anyway. Every step becomes more deliberate, and he realizes the Bridge is helping to re-center him.

He looks over the edge, which entices him to get down on his hands and knees and gaze into the water. How deep is it? Are there any Fish or Turtles swimming around down there? What about Leeches?

With some apprehension, he dangles his feet in the water, which feels refreshingly cool. There he sits, for what seems like a long time, even though he has no particular reason for doing so. It just feels good to relax and let his mind wander along with his eyes.

The Last Sojourn: Healing by Fire

Sarah awaits Chris as he comes off of the Bridge. "While you were sitting there," she said, "you reminded me of something Albert Einstein said: 'Look deep, deep into nature, and then you will understand everything better.'"

"Especially myself and where I come from," Chris replies.

Sarah nods, with a reassuring smile.

"You've now come full circle," she continues. "Right up ahead, the Trail takes a sharp right and brings you back to the Threshold Bridge. But first, I'd like to take you to a place where you can sit in council with Earth, Air, Fire, and Water. There, Nature speaks loud and clear. At the same time, you'll be able to see and hear in the distance reminders of the modern life you'll be going back to. It'll give you the opportunity to bring it all together: your past, your experience here, and the life you'll be walking back into."

Taking a short side Trail, the two of them round a bend and step into an opening overlooking a tree-ringed pond. Off to the west, Chris can see a couple of buildings. In front of him is a fire ring surrounded by log benches. He sits down and wonders how many people like him and how many groups with their therapist-guides have sat here before him, staring into the flames while reflecting on their Trail experiences.

"The voices that have spoken to you will go on speaking, wherever you are," says Sarah. "All you have to do is keep listening to them."

"Easier said than done," Chris replies. "In just my short time here I can see where immersion in Nature helps get to the essence of communication. But what about after I leave?"

"The essence of communication is what many Native people call Truthspeaking. You've experienced the essence here— you've Truthspoken—as it's all about spontaneity and listening. How you speak your Truth is just as important. I think it was Franklin Delano Roosevelt who said, 'Be sincere; be brief; be seated.' If you can do that, you're halfway there. The other half, of course, is listening. You can be spontaneous and listen—that is, Truthspeak—anywhere."

"Maybe *you* can."

"And so can you. Buddha said that three things cannot be long hidden: the sun, the moon, and the Truth. I'll give you a clue for how you can find hidden Truth anywhere: enter the stillness. Then just embrace the naked Truth for what it is. Any words we try to put to Truth end up being only a bad translation. That's why Roosevelt said, 'Be brief.'"

"Again," Chris replies with more than a hint of frustration, "I'm not in Nature all the time like you are. Let's be real; I need something that works for me back in the city. Otherwise, I'm afraid I'll end up right back where I started."

77

"It is said that the only sin is separation," replies Sarah. "The only thing that separates you from Nature is the illusion of separation that your mind creates. Remember, you are Nature's child wherever you go; and Nature is everywhere, even though we may have cleverly disguised it. This includes us. No matter what we do, say, think, or feel, our inner nature is still Nature."

"I get it. It's my state of mind, not my state of place, that separates me from Nature."

"That's it! One reason it's so important to have a clear state of mind is so you can listen to the stillness. Nature can then bring you to the layer of honesty you thrive best at in any given moment. There are times when it's vital to recognize that love and hate are the same core emotion, and that there is no difference between praise and criticism. In the stillness, there are no words or beliefs to distinguish between them."

Taken aback by the profundity of his sharing with Sarah, Chris remembers the Token he picked up at the Welcome Center. He gently and reverently takes the Token from his pocket and holds the icon in cupped hands. Tears come to Chris's eyes as he realizes how much strength and support the Token has contributed to his healing mission.

The Dance of Remembering and Forgetting

After a few minutes, Sarah sits beside Chris and says in a voice barely above a whisper, "Hippocrates once said that Nature cures—not the physician. Yet for Nature to cure, we need to not only listen, but remember.

"However, we need a way to remember that is lasting and not subject to the whims of our fickle thoughts and feelings. To understand how to accomplish that, we need to look at the three parts of our brain: the *reptilian*, which manages reproduction and basic body functions; the *mammalian*, which is the seat of our emotions and long-term memories; and the *primate*, which is responsible for our rational processes. It's the mammalian brain's long-term memory that we want to access, which we can do with the shamanic technique of fire-induced trance."

"Why fire?" Chris asks. "And why trance?"

"Because fire is what made us human. Around a half-million years ago, our distant ancestors tamed fire, which allowed them to prepare the high-energy foods needed to support our evolving brains. You'll notice that all other animals fear fire, yet we are drawn to it. This special relationship we have with fire is the doorway to the deeper reaches of our minds that shamans have been using as a healing tool for time immemorial. Trance is simply the state of consciousness we dwell in when we are centered in our mammalian minds. To enter trance, you just have to sit before a fire and let your ancestral memories guide you."

The Dragon's Breath

"What you're doing is becoming *the Dragon's Breath*," says Sarah as she helps Chris start a Fire. "As I'm sure you know, Dragons are formidable symbols in our folklore. Since ancient times, they've been one of shamans' most potent spirit helpers. In the East, they're known to bring growth and good fortune; and in the European tradition, they help with clarity and the ability to overcome adversity. That's the Dragon's Breath."

"Hmm ...interesting. But how does that help my healing?"

"Fire is the Dragon's Breath, and Fire transforms. It's one of the most potent vehicles for change. A fallen tree branch takes years—maybe decades—to break down into soil, yet Fire does it in a matter of minutes. Think of a decomposing branch as burning slowly. The same byproducts—carbon dioxide, water, and minerals—are produced as when a tree burns, only at a much slower rate. It's the same with healing, and that's why Fire—the Dragon's Breath—is such a powerful and favored transformational tool for shamans."

"That makes sense," Chris replies, "but I don't get the connection between sitting in front of a Fire and becoming the Dragon's Breath."

"When you breathe," explains Sarah, "you engage in the same slow-burning process as the decomposing branch—you're breaking down food into carbon dioxide, water, and minerals. The same thing happens on a healing level when you use Conscious Breathing. Now imagine what breathing Fire could do to rev it up!"

"Here's how it's done: when the Fire flares up, inhale; then exhale between flareups. Take a deep breath when the Fire surges, and breathe shallow when the Fire wanes. Let the Fire's rhythm tell you how fast or slow to breathe. Before you know it, the Fire will have you naturally breathing in sync with it—you'll have become the Dragon's Breath."

Sarah then steps back to let Chris gaze into the flames. Before long, their leaping and swaying seduces him into a trance state. Everything he heard, saw, and felt on the Trail comes back to him, and it merges with everything he brought with him. In that instant, there is no more separation. He is no longer the victim of his past, nor is he above what happened then. He accepts, and he embraces.

Letting-Go Rituals

As the Fire fades to embers, Chris comes back to the iridescent Dragonflies darting over the pond and the soft breeze twitching the needles on the nearby branches. He lets out a long satisfied sigh as he realizes that he just imprinted what he gained here into his long-term memory.

Taking a pencil and a piece of paper from the box he sees sitting beside his bench, Chris writes down what he'd like to release, then thoughtfully lays the folded paper on the embers.

As his old fears, regrets, and judgments take flame, Chris watches the smoke rise into the ethers. "I have released myself of my burden," he tells himself, "and I have done it in a way that will not contaminate others." He feels good as he watches the golden flames transform his woundedness into bright energy and clean ash that the flowers and trees will convert to fresh aromatic essences that will support the healing of others.

He then holds the Medicine Stick in front of him that Sarah suggested he carry with him on the Trail. The Stick becomes a repository for his grief as all the memories of past relationships flood through him. The flames help him see that those people left because of his woundedness, not because of their failings. Chris starts sobbing uncontrollably, and Sarah gently comforts him.

After he catches his breath, she leads him in taking several deeper, clearing breaths, which help relax him. She then suggests that he break the stick in two as a symbol of breaking the grief.

He reverently places the pieces on the coals and watches them smolder. He is glad they don't immediately burst into flame, as the thick, ropey smoke that rises from them draws forth the old memories one more time. He takes the opportunity to express his gratitude for those beautiful people who graced his life and taught him about himself.

Bringing It Home

Chris feels complete as he crosses the Threshold Bridge. It's been a long time since he's felt so good about returning home. With what he's gained—and with what he's left behind—he knows his life can be different from here onward.

"You've done some tremendous work today," says Sarah.

He can't help but smile and feel good about that. At the same time, he knows that there is much more walk ahead. "What can I do to keep on track?" he asks.

"Let's stop at the Cairn on the way out," she replies. "There might be a Crystal or a Burl that speaks to you there. If so, take it home and place it where it'll be a regular reminder of what Nature gifted you here. You can take your Token home with you also.

"But mostly, it's what you carry inside, and how you keep it alive. Have you heard the saying that there's nobody like an old fool, because there's no substitute for experience? Fortunately, experience works both ways. If I could give you only one piece of advice, I'd ask you to remember that we become what we surround ourselves with. It's the easiest way to change and stay on the Healing Path: just hang out with the people you want to emulate.

"And you can do what many others find helpful: come back and Walk the Trail again. For some, it's a renewal of what they gained; others call it a retreat or pilgrimage. Some folks who live in the area stop by often, even if it's to just Walk one of the Labyrinths. Others come annually, sometimes on the anniversary of their first Walk.

"I know you live some distance away. You can take a Remote Walk whenever you like. You could put on a recording of Nature sounds, then envision you are Walking the Trail, or sitting in your Comfort Spot." (See chapter 14 for more on Remote Walking.)

For Gratitude: The Trail's End Feast

"There is one more thing you can do to keep your Walk alive in your heart. Did you know that every culture, in every era, civilized or aboriginal, typically marks the conclusion of rites of passage, rituals, and healings with a Feast? It's the same in our society. Have you ever been to a wedding, funeral, anniversary, graduation, or just about any other significant event, without there being a formal meal?"

"I never thought of it that way," Chris replies, "but you're right. There's something about a banquet, or even the main meal at Grandma's house when we have a family reunion, that brings us all together. Everybody seems to be in a good mood and lots of stories and memories are shared."

"Believe it or not," says Sarah, "it's the body-mind connection again. Sharing food is Grounding; it fosters relaxation and goodwill, and it strengthens relationships. And as you noted, recalling old memories helps connect past with present."

"I know it was suggested on the packing list that I bring food, and bring enough to share if I had a Guide. Is what you're talking about the reason for that?"

"Yes; that and more. It started for you at home already. The whole ritual of procuring, preparing, and packing the food is a metaphor for preparing to have the healing gifts of Nature feed your inner hunger for healing.

"With our healing ritual completed, you and I can now have our Feast of Gratitude, for all that you have been gifted, and for the honor it has been for me to serve you. In the tradition we follow here, which has been passed down to us from the Native elders, we begin the Feast by placing a bit of each food in the Fire, in remembrance of those who have come before us. This includes our ancestors, and those whose footsteps we followed on this Trail.

"As we take our first bite, let's think of the enrichment we gained from the Journey we just completed. Think of Mother Nature, who has given us the food that nourishes both our bodies and our hearts. Then let us follow Rumi's advice, when he said, 'Gratitude is the wine of the soul. Go ahead, get drunk!'"

For Renewal: The Commemorative Feast

"What you say doesn't just make sense," Chris replies, "I can *feel* it. I wish there was some way I could take this Trail's End Feast home with me—I know it would help me stay on track with my healing."

"Do you know how birthdays and wedding anniversaries help in renewing vows and resolutions? You can do the same thing, by holding Commemorative Feasts of your Trail Walk. Invite your friends or family to the Feast, and share the story of your Walk with them.

"It might seem strange to have a Commemorative Feast with people who didn't share the experience with you. Yet your Healing Journey is the Healing Journey of those close to you, whether or not they realize it. That's the law of attraction that we mentioned a bit back: your wellness becomes their wellness.

"The same is true for those who follow in your footsteps, both literally on this Trail and in your life. For that reason, some people see the Commemorative Feast as not only support for them, but a responsibility to others."

The Healing Camp Deep in Nature

While Chris and Sarah break bread together, she tells him the story of another enchanted health-giving refuge. "It's down a spur off the far end of the Healing Nature Trail that you'd notice only if it was pointed out to you. It takes you off of the island and into the wilds beyond.

"After a half mile, the Path ends at a camp that harkens back to the time when bark, thatch, and rawhide were the preferred building materials. Two wigwams, an arbor, and a lean-to perch on a ridge overlooking a pond teeming with Water Lilies, Chorus Frogs, and Waterfowl. Kamgabwequay, one of our Ojibwe Elders, named the camp *Mashkodens*, which means *Little Prairie*, after the Blueberry Meadow that rolls down from the ridge. "It's there at Mashkodens that therapists bring groups for in-depth Nature-based therapy. The camp is also available for group Breathwork sessions, yoga, and other therapies. And when the camp isn't reserved for other purposes, it's available for individual and group retreats."

Sarah goes on to say that practitioners and retreatants are drawn to Mashkodens for the feeling of intimacy with Nature that it offers. "There's the smell of a wood Fire, the essence of pine from the bough mat around the hearth, the chortle of Ravens overhead, and the serenading of Frogs just a few paces away. If you're quiet, Deer venture out on the meadow in plain sight. In the evening, Coyotes and Owls give concerts. Wolves, Bears, and Bobcats sometimes venture close to camp, yet it's the rare person who sees one. They're shy and typically disappear at the first sign of humans. What you do see, though, is an array of Wildflowers, Birds, and Butterflies, with Chipmunks scampering at your feet and wild berries tempting you in their season."

"It sounds like a fairytale place," Chris responds. "I can only imagine that in such an openly inviting setting, there has to be healing."

"You're right; that's what nearly everybody tells us. And that's why I'd like to suggest that you book your stay at Mashkodens well in advance, to be sure you get your preferred date."

Find Healing Nature Anywhere

"There's one more thing I'd like to leave with you," says Sarah. "Now that you've Walked the Trail, you know that the magic is not in the Trail per se, but rather in who the Trail introduces you to. And you can find Her everywhere, once you know what to look for. A walk in any city park, along any waterway, or through any patch of trees, grass, or scrub, can be turned into a Healing Nature Walk. Even though it doesn't have all the features of a certified Healing Nature Trail, you'll still be caressed in her caring embrace. Her essence is there—her Aromatherapy, her Grounding energy, her guiding voices.

"Other features you're looking for are likely there as well, though they may not be as obvious as on a Healing Nature Trail. Let's say you want a Reflective Nook or a Panoramic Vista. Reflect on what it brings you, then look around you for the place that will do it. Be careful not to get hung up on the envisionment of the actual Nook or Vista, but rather relive the *experience* you had there. Then you might notice that what you're looking for is already there before you, only in a form that you didn't recognize.

"Another way to help a healing feature materialize is to read about it in the *Forest Bathing Companion* or *Healing Nature Trail* books. Take note of its basic characteristics, rather than its visual description, and you might then watch it take shape in front of you, wherever you are. Like all mothers, Nature usually finds a way to give us what we need."

Farewell

It's time for Chris to leave. He gives Sarah a long hug—it's the only way he can say goodbye. Though it's not like him to be at a loss for something to say, Chris realizes that the world Sarah opened up for him goes beyond words.

"I understand," says Sarah softly. "Please feel free to contact me after you've had some time to sit with all of this. Otherwise, I'll be in touch with you anyway to check in on how you're doing, and to work with you on integrating what you've awakened to here today.

"Right now, why don't you just take some time for yourself. The gate swings both ways, by the way; so you might want to Walk the Labyrinth again before you hit the road. Or you could go lay up on the Cosmorinth and let everything percolate for a bit. On the other hand, you might just want to relax at one of the picnic tables near the parking area. Whichever option you choose, it's a good way to transition back into the world out there."

First Chris heads for the Welcome Center to check out and leave a donation. And he wants to get a book or two that caught his eye on the way in. Sarah suggested that he pick up some Balsam Fir essential oil so he can continue Aromatherapy and body-mind connectedness on his own.

That's all fine and good, Chris thinks, *but the main reason I want to take some of that Northwoodsy smelling oil home with me is to bring back memories of this dreamy day I just spent in another world.*

While in the Welcome Center, Chris notices a large print of the Threshold Bridge that speaks to him. A copy goes home with him to hang in his living room, but not only for its beauty. He wants it to remind him of the span there once was between his life and the serenity of Nature, and of how he bridged that span to bring the two together.

Before leaving, Chris writes a few words in the guestbook for those who come after him. The cover of the guestbook reads:

Dear Journeyer,

We hope you had a rich and rewarding time
here at the Healing Nature Center.
We invite you to share something of your experience
in this notebook—a new awareness,
a special moment, or anything else you like.

Along with us, other guests
would like to hear about your time here.
What you leave of yourself on these pages
may inspire others, and maybe help someone
surmount a hurdle.

We are deeply grateful for the time
you spent with us here in the Cradle of Nature,
and we want you to know that you have a place here
—you are always welcome back.

We wish you safe travels
and an ever-enriching Healing Journey.

PART TWO

NATURE'S HEALING TOUCH

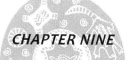

CHAPTER NINE

Breathing and Grounding with Trees

"The physician treats, but nature heals," said Greek physician Hippocrates, who is known as the father of medicine. In this chapter we explore the many and wondrous ways that plants, animals, Earth, Water, Fire, and the very Air we breathe, bring us to wellness. Full descriptions of the following healing features of Nature, along with additional techniques and applications, can be found in the companion book, *The Healing Nature Trail: Forest Bathing for Recovery and Awakening.*

Breathing in Nature

Breath is life—not only our life but that of our mother planet and our entire solar system. Perhaps you weren't aware of the fact that our solar system breathes. Our planet and all of her sibling celestial bodies are awash in a continuous flow of charged particles that the sun exhales. Without it, our planet would have no life.

Our Earth breathes by bringing nourishing carbon dioxide to the plants, which they convert to oxygen and exhale as a waste product. In turn, we animals make the plants' breath our breath by inhaling it—which to us is life-giving oxygen. We then exhale our waste product, carbon dioxide, which the plants inhale.

This is Breathing in Nature: all of Life sharing one breath.

Finding Nature's Breath

The Healing Nature Trail experience is centered on Conscious Breathing. It can add depth and dimension to nearly every Trail-related practice. Think of Conscious Breathing as feeling. Nature comes alive when we mindfully breathe with her. Sharing the same breath with the animals brings us all the closer to sharing the same language. Conscious Breathing strengthens the body-mind connection and energizes the healing process. This form of breathing can take us deep into our subconscious selves and encourage what lies there to surface.

Conscious Breathing as it is practiced and taught on Healing Nature Trails traces its origins back to what the author learned from the practices of indigenous cultures, and directly from Nature. In his words:

> I first became aware of breathing rhythms when I was child watching wild animals. Often the only movement I could detect from them was their breathing. When a Dove was frightened by a Hawk passing overhead, she would huff, then momentarily hold her breath. A Fox slowly stalking a Pheasant would freeze, and his breathing would become slow, shallow, and spaced as accurately as if guided by a metronome. Wanting to remain invisible, a frightened Rabbit would crouch in the grass, yet his twitching nose and vibrating sides caused by his rapid breathing could be detected by a sharp eye.
>
> Over time, I learned to read animals' breathing to the point where it often told me what they were feeling, thinking, and doing. That ability helped me integrate into the Wolf pack I lived with for several years when I was a young adult. Wolves, who are social beings like us, have complex personalities. I had to learn their often-silent language, which was based on nuances of facial expression, posture, tail/ruff positioning, and variances in breathing. Whoofs, pants, quick exhales, and short, sharp inhales each had their own meanings, which were elaborated upon by the way they were executed.

Shortly after I left the pack, I was taught more about Conscious Breathing by the Ojibwe, Menominee, Hopi, Blackfoot, Iroquois, and Lakota elders with whom I apprenticed. I learned the benefits of breathing through the nose by holding mouthfuls of water for extended periods of time while doing other activities.

The most demanding—and rewarding—lesson came from having to run with a mouthful of water. In order to maintain the blood oxygen level I needed to keep me going, I had no choice but to make every breath count as much as possible. It's hard to pant through your nose, especially for any period of time, so I had to slowly inhale and breathe deeply, to completely, fully, fill my lungs. Then I had to exhale completely, to make room for the next full breath. I found that as my technique improved, I slowed my breathing even more, as it kept me better oxygenated than did short, partial inhales.

In time, I naturally fell into a rhythm where I took full, deep inhales, all the way down to the bottom of my lungs, which were followed by full and complete exhales.

Makwa Giizis, the Ojibwe elder who guided me on my Vision Quest (a rite of passage into adulthood where one fasts alone in the wilderness to find your life's direction), showed me how to breathe with trees. "Go to the Elder Tree who calls for you," he would say. "Wrap your arms around her. Hug her close and feel her heartbeat. Breathe into her bark, and she will breathe with you."

"'What did she tell you?' he would ask when I came back.

When I had nothing much to say, he would encourage me to "Go back and breathe with her. Then listen."

From there, I came to feel the heartbeat of the Forest, and I started to breathe spontaneously in sync with its pulse. Thanks to my childhood training in animal observation, I came to realize that all the other creatures were doing the same. Like clouds parting from the sun, it one day dawned on me that we all shared the same breath! Even more so, I realized that breath wasn't just giving me life; breath *was* life.

Breath for Healing

Just as *Healing Nature* is a double entendre (we help Nature heal as she helps us heal), so is *Breathing in Nature*: we inhale Nature's healing essences while we are immersed in Nature. Twenty-five hundred years ago, the Buddha elaborated on this double meaning for *Breathing in Nature* when he said, "There is a most wonderful way to help overcome directly grief and sorrow, end pain and anxiety. One remains established in the observation of the feelings of the body and of the mind by going to the forest, to the foot of a tree, sitting down and holding one's body straight, and establishing mindfulness. By breathing in, one is aware of breathing in. Breathing out, one is aware of breathing out. Breathing in, I am aware of my whole body. Breathing out, I am aware of my whole body. Breathing in, I calm the activities of my body. Breathing out, I calm the activities of my body."

Conscious Breathing in Nature may be the most accessible and easy-to-use healing modality. Our breath is always with us, we are always using it, and we can channel it for an intended purpose at any time. A tree to breathe under, as the Buddha and Makwa Giizis suggest, is usually not too far away.

A Short Course in Conscious Breathing

All you need to do is find a quiet place, where there is just you and your breath.

Step One: Connect with Your Breath

Relax, then inhale, imagining that you are taking your first breath. Feel it coming in through your nose, then back out through your nose. Is it cool or is it warm? Can you hear it? Smell it? What are your chest and gut doing? Are you breathing fast or slow? Do you pause between breaths? Does your head move when you breathe?

Now envision that you have become your breath, going in and out, in one continuous motion. Let your breath take you where it will—into your body, your blood, your muscles, your mind. It is your Guide for this Journey.

Feel your feet, solidly rooted. Let your breath travel down the length of your body, through your knees and calves and out through your feet, straight into the ground. With every exhale, your breath flows through every organ and muscle—through your very bones—in a continual stream into the Earth.

Step Two: Establish Circular Breathing

1. Breathe a bit faster than normal for the situation.
2. Balance your inhale and exhale by giving equal time and presence to both. Count if you need to.
3. Let your inhale flow into your exhale, so there is no interruption between them.
4. Imagine your inhale coming up your spine, your exhale flowing down your chest, and your inhale again rising up your spine, in a circular fashion.

As goes the breath, so goes the body. When you breathe in a circular fashion, your senses keen and you become present within your body. Your mind grows vibrant and active, processing and synthesizing the increased input. You feel ready for anything or nothing.

Step Three: Create a Rolling Breath

1. Inhale into your gut.
2. Continue the inhale by expanding into your chest.
3. At the top of your inhale, let your chest relax and contract.
4. Your gut will follow, then seamlessly begin to expand with your next inhale.

After a few breaths, the rhythm should start to come naturally, as this is the typical way we breathe when we are centered, relaxed, and in good physical shape. It's called *Rolling Breath* because of the rolling motion of the gut and chest as they go in and out. Rolling Breath enlivens your senses, prepares your lungs and metabolism to absorb the healing essences of Nature, and strengthens and stimulates your internal organs.

Step Four: Integrate Your Breathing

Here you merge your breathing seamlessly with whatever you are doing so that it can serve without distracting or interfering. To others, your Conscious Breathing should become invisible.

This synching of breath and movement tends to happen naturally. Have you noticed your tendency to inhale when something stimulating or shocking occurs, then exhale when it's over? We see this reflected in the sayings "It took my breath away," "It's a breathtaking view," and "It helped me breathe easy."

As you become practiced at integrating your breathing, you will likely find it easily falling into sync with the sway of the trees, movements of the animals, and the general rhythm of the life around you. You will be moving with them by breathing with them.

Plying the Body-Mind Connection

The Healing Nature Trail is one of many bridges, bends, and benches. Transitions from one habitat type to another are common on the Trail. So are small footbridges without railings, which—even though they're only a step or two above ground level—can create a slight sense of uneasiness and have you crossing with caution.

The entire Trail, in fact, keeps you on your toes. There are numerous sharp turns, small changes in elevation, variations in topography, and forks in the Trail. The walking surface varies as well, going from sod to pine needles to boardwalk to wood shavings.

The same is true of the Labyrinths. The Gateway Labyrinth has fourteen switchbacks, and there are endless potential turns in the Zen Untangle, Cosmorinth, and Aquarinth. Add the several styles of Finger Labyrinth and the Zen Garden to the mix, and you have a total experience designed to keep you present, attuned, and challenged.

As Goes the Body, so Goes the Mind

The body-mind connection is so strong that each of the functional readjustments you make creates a parallel shift in your mind. When you change direction on the Trail, you open up the possibility for a mental change of direction. When you step off the main Path to take a side fork, you make it all the more likely that you'll be able to explore other possibilities for your life.

In addition, suppressed thoughts and feelings find the opportunity to emerge and be cleared. Outmoded patterns of behavior that you were previously blind to can be recognized. The ego is encouraged to follow suit and relax self-protective boundaries, which increases your state of presence. Feeling more yourself, you have the wherewithal to abandon your conventional relational modus operandi and open yourself to new possibilities.

With virtually every feature of the Trail, the designers took its potential effect on the body- mind connection into consideration. They knew that there is no easier or more effective way to create avenues for psycho-emotional change than by creating literal avenues for changing up the physical self. Altogether, these Trail features create a continual-movement change-up, with the cumulative effect building in the mind the further you progress on the Trail. Along with that, your ego's efforts to resist change progressively weaken.

Eventually the old saying, "As goes the body, so goes the mind," proves to be true. If you are like most people, at some point on your Trail Walk you will start to experience a surprising sense of mind-expanding openness, along with a flood of considerations and feelings that you didn't know you were capable of. A little further down the Trail, fresh perspectives might take shape around old experiences, and new possibilities could come to light. If you are on the Trail because of trauma, the newfound sense of self you gain can make your Healing Journey look not quite so scary.

Grounding in Nature

"It was good for the skin to touch the bare Earth," said Oglala Lakota chief Luther Standing Bear. "The old people liked to remove their moccasins and walk with their bare feet on the sacred Earth …They sat on the ground with the feeling of being close to a mothering power. The soil was soothing, strengthening, cleansing, and healing."

Standing Bear's people were practicing what is now commonly called "Grounding." It involves direct skin contact with the surface of the Earth. Along with sensory contact, Grounding connects us with the Earth's electrical field. Direct contact with the Earth grounds our bodies, inducing favorable electro-physiological and psycho-emotional changes that promote optimum health.

Many people use the terms "Earthing," and "Barefooting" synonymously with "Grounding," yet we prefer the latter, as it carries the double meaning of becoming grounded in both yourself and Earth energy.

Research has found that Grounding yields positive health benefits to such an extent that it has been called "electric nutrition." It has been found to boost the human immune response by minimizing inflammation and accelerating wound recovery. The practice enhances sleep quality, balances cortisol levels, activates the parasympathetic nervous system, and reduces pain and stress, among other health benefits. Grounding may be the most effective, essential, affordable, and accessible antioxidant there is.

Grounding can be accomplished in a number of ways—with the hands or feet, lying flat on your back or face down, sitting, kneeling, crawling, or through artificial methods involving electrical conduction.

Grounding on the Trail

Visitors are encouraged to Walk barefoot if they are able to do so and if weather permits. Along with the therapeutic effects, Walking barefoot or with minimal footwear promotes healthy feet and legs, along with good posture.

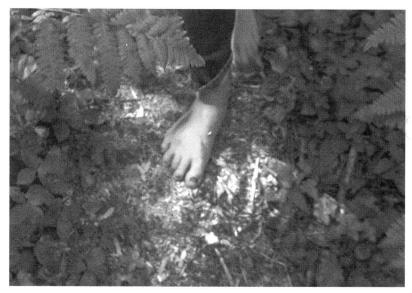

Grounding in Earth's healing energy

Though some weather conditions are more conducive to Grounding than others, the regenerative effects of the practice can be experienced in any weather. Dampness of any form increases conductivity, with Walking barefoot in the rain giving the strongest connection. Exposing some of your skin to the rain enhances the experience even more. Snow is a moderate insulator from Grounding energy, yet there is typically enough of a benefit to make a Trail Walk worthwhile.

The Grounding experience on the Trails can be amplified in these ways:

▶ Embrace an Elder Tree or spend extra time sitting beneath her, with your back resting against her.

▶ Lie down on the ground, anywhere along the Trail that is open, out of the way, and does not harm vegetation. You'll experience the fringe benefit of increased sensory awareness.

▶ Practice the *Rooting* exercise found later in this chapter.

Along the Trails you'll find benches periodically spaced for rest and reflection. People who are not able to sit on the ground or Walk the entire Trail due to injury, mobility impairment, or other reasons, can rest on a bench and Ground themselves there.

Some Trails have benches made of large-diameter log sections lying directly on the ground. Their mass and substance make them effective conductors of the Earth's Grounding energy. Those not able to sit or lie directly on the forest floor can then Ground themselves by sitting on these special benches. When a bench sits adjacent to a tree, resting one's back on the tree increases the Grounding effect.

Shamanic Grounding

Healing Nature Guides follow in the tradition of Shamanic practitioners by helping facilitate a client's Grounding experience. Prior to the Trail Walk, Guides interview their clients, to determine what type of Grounding would best serve their needs:

▶ Barefoot or light footwear?

▶ Over all or particular parts of the Trail?

▶ Sitting, lying, or crawling?

▶ Incorporating a Grounding ritual, such as *Rooting* (found later in chapter)?

In shamanic traditions around the world, a more advanced form of Grounding that involves full-body immersion is practiced, for both physical and psycho-emotional healing purposes. Earth, water, and vegetation are the most common covering mediums. The rituals are known by various names, such as *Toltec Earth Embrace*, *Burial Extraction*, *Ritual of the Sacred Burial*, the *Death Rebirth Ritual*, and *Earth Swaddling*.

Full-immersion Grounding is a powerful transformative technique that should be practiced only under the guidance of a seasoned shamanic practitioner. Without proper preparation and oversight, a person risks psychic overload and physical harm. If a Healing Nature Guide or other healthcare practitioner is trained in Full Immersion Grounding and receives prior approval from the Center Director, the ritual can be practiced as part of the Trail Walk experience.

Rooting: An Exercise for Stronger Connection

Grounding occurs spontaneously when Walking barefoot or with minimal footwear, or when sitting/lying on the earth. Yet the experience can be magnified with various practices. A very effective one that can be used nearly anywhere is called *Rooting*. Here's how it is done:

1. **Find a quiet, shaded place** with sparse ground vegetation, preferably in a grove of elder trees, amongst boulders, or in a recessed area such as a depression or ravine.

2. **Remove footwear** you may be wearing (weather permitting), so that your feet can be in direct contact with the earth.

3. **Spread your feet** to the width of your shoulders and stand with knees slightly bent.

4. **Relax your eyes** and let them partially close so that you are looking softly and not focusing on anything. Let your eyes close if they so choose.

5. **Breathe slowly and consciously,** following the guidance found earlier in this chapter.

6. **Continue until you feel rooted.** A deep calm will come over you, and you may experience a slight tingling sensation. Go no longer than half an hour.

7. **End with several deep inhales** and long, slow exhales. Then gently continue your Walk.

If you do not feel any change, it may be because you were already Rooted. Otherwise, you can Root more strongly by resting your back against an embankment, rock face, elder tree, or by finding a location more conducive to Rooting.

Water Grounding

Native people hold Water sacred. It is the blood of Mother Earth, essential to all life; and it is one of the four sacred elements, along with Earth, Air, and Fire. Water plays a central role in the cleansing and healing rituals of many cultures. Purification through ablution (the washing of hands and sacred vessels) is an essential component of Islamic prayer rituals, Baptism by water is a traditional Christian practice, and the Seven Sacred Rivers are central to Hindu practice. Like most American Indians, the Ojibwe people of northern Wisconsin hold Sweat Lodge Ceremonies, where water plays a central healing and cleansing role.

We can become Grounded in ourselves and in Earth energy most viscerally through water immersion, which is commonly referred to as *Water Grounding*. It provides an amplified Grounding experience because the human organism is itself mostly water, developed *in utero* in an aquatic environment, and lives on a planet whose surface is 71 percent water. Serving as a longstanding healing modality for indigenous peoples, Water Immersion is growing as a form of therapy and recreation in modern cultures.

Water Immersion has been found to induce relaxation, lower anxiety, improve memory, and increase focus, along with balancing out serotonin—the feel-good neurotransmitter. Depression, chronic fatigue, and cancer treatments may be successfully augmented with water immersion.

A Healing Nature Guide who is trained in the practical and ritual aspects of the practice can incorporate it into a Trail Walk with prior approval from the Center Director.

CHAPTER TEN

How Labyrinths, Plants, and Animals Speak to Us

In this day, not many people are familiar with Labyrinths. A few of us know about the Labyrinths of medieval cathedrals and courtyards, or the classical Labyrinths of ancient times. Most of us who know about Labyrinths came upon them as children in the form of mazes. Our childhood activity books had them, in the form of a tangle of trails, with dead ends and looming danger that we had to find our way through in order to get to a buried treasure or escape from a castle dungeon.

Labyrinths have made a comeback. They are helping transform the lives of many people across Europe and the Americas, and they figure prominently in the Healing Nature Trail experience.

In Walking a Labyrinth, one circles around its center until reaching it, then spirals out in reverse until returning to the beginning point. The ritual stands on its own as a circumambulation practice, and it is found as a component of many other traditions, from ancient Middle Eastern and Scandinavian to medieval cathedrals to Native cultures in the southwestern United States.

The Labyrinths of classical times were constructed and used for these reasons:

- As divining mediums, often in conjunction with the astrological courses of celestial bodies.
- To prepare for battle or a long Journey.
- To atone for sins or escape karma and the cycle of reincarnation.

- As a symbolic pilgrimage, stroll through an enchanted forest, or Walk on the Path of Life.
- To attain clarity or find relief from suffering.
- A vehicle to progress from numbness to awakening, or from the secular to the sacred.

Here are the most common reasons Healing Nature Trail Walkers give for using Labyrinths:

- Curiosity
- A pilgrimage
- A refuge
- Walking Meditation
- An Inward Journey
- Unwinding mental and emotional entanglements
- Stress release
- Deep trauma work
- Life-transition support

Many of us feel the increasing need for self-reflection and simplifying our lives. We yearn to live with a greater sense of wellness and fulfillment. The drive to reunite our minds, bodies, and spirits may be even stronger for us than it was for people in times past.

In our quest, some of us find that the therapeutic and spiritual techniques of our ancestors are just as pertinent today as they were back then. This may explain the resurgence of interest in Labyrinths, and why we are still able to experience their benefits, even though we no longer live in cultures where Labyrinths are commonly used.

The Four Stages of Walking a Labyrinth

First: Preparation

Before setting foot on the Sinuous Path, take a moment to go over this list:

1. Take a few deep, conscious breaths, to immerse yourself in the now.

2. Let go of expectations and relax into the experience.

3. Sensitize yourself by observing your surroundings, listening, and touching.

4. Go at your own pace. You can pass others and be passed.

5. Stay present with whatever emerges and breathe through it.

6. Take nothing literally. Everything is a symbol or metaphor for something deeper.

Second: The Inward Journey

As we enter a Labyrinth, we symbolically leave behind the pressures and stresses that so often keep us from the inner work—and mask the awarenesses—necessary for healing and personal evolution. Each bend of the Path strips away more of the world as we know it; more of who we *think* we are. In essence, we are ritually killing our old self.

We then stand alone, stripped down to our essential self. Before us lies the Hero's Journey. Shadow surrounds us, and the Void awaits to engulf us, perhaps on the next step, or the next. All we have to guide us through is reflection and nebulous voices.

Third: Entering the Womb

Out of the shadow emerges the sacred destination at the very center of the Meander. There awaits the Minotaur: the bastard spawn of our fragmented self. We must defeat (i.e., embrace and consume) the abominable beast in order to be reborn into ourselves.

Now is the time for Conscious Breathing, to imbue our new self with the Breath of Life. The first breath is for awakening, the second breath is for illumination, and the following breaths are for meditative listening.

We stay in the Womb until we feel complete and ready to enter the Birth Canal.

Fourth: The Return Journey

When we retrace our steps, we find that nothing looks the same from the backside as it did from the front. What was fragmented is now becoming integrated; what was disturbing has somehow become insightful.

As we Walk the serpentine Path from birth to spreading our new wings before the fresh breeze that greets us at the Labyrinth's threshold, we use the time to integrate all that we have gained. Following are the potential benefits of that integration:

- Mental clarity
- Reduced stress and anxiety
- Revitalized sense of intuition
- Improved state of well-being
- Expanded self-awareness and capacity for self-reflection
- The aptitude for Trance Journeying

All Healing Nature Trails offer one or more Labyrinthine Experience options. The original Trail in Three Lakes, Wisconsin, USA, has seven different types of Labyrinths threaded out along the Trail like a string of pearls: a Gateway Turf Labyrinth, a Cosmorinth, a Stump Labyrinth, an Aquarinth, a Zen Untangle, a Zen Garden Labyrinth, and handheld Finger Labyrinths.

The Language of Plants and Animals

Indigenous hunter-gatherers the world round refer to the animals and plants they live with as their sisters and brothers. This is not just a platitude, or some hollow religious belief. These people live in community with the plants and animals, where they rely on each other for their sustenance and welfare. In doing so, they come to know each other intimately. They live together in honor and respect, as true kin. When Native people call a Frog "Little Brother" or a Tree "Grandmother," they mean it literally.

With such an interdependent relationship, the humans, the other animals, and the plants get to know each other well. They come to know each other's needs and desires. They talk amongst themselves, asking each other for favors, and complaining when things don't go well. They communicate in the universal language, which is known by many as *Naturespeak* (as mentioned in chapter 4).

Here is where some people get derailed. Nearly everyone agrees that at least rudimentary communication is possible between us and "higher" animals, such as the great apes and cetaceans. And many of us have spoken with Dogs, Cats, or Horses. But a Snake? Or a Cricket? Even better, when have you last met someone who has carried on a conversation with Grass or a Bush?

Plant Sentience

Peoples of many cultures throughout the ages have held trees in high esteem. Their presence imparts a sense of comfort and protection, and Walking amongst them uplifts the spirit. Since time immemorial, people have gone into the forests to seek sanctuary, take retreats, and commune with the ethereal.

Classic Norse, Celtic, Hindu, Egyptian, and American Indian cultures recognized the life-giving power of trees, as witnessed by their legends and religious texts. Buddhist scriptures describe the unlimited kindness of trees, how they give generously and offer protection to all beings. Traditional legends and Native elders have elaborated on these relationships. Here, however, let's review how modern science is helping us reconnect with our innate knowledge of plants, and with the Legends about our relationship with them.

One reason for our distant relationship with plants is that we consider them to be lower life forms than animals, and much lower than us humans. We see this perspective reflected in our beliefs and daily practices. We mow the grass without thought for countless plants we are tearing limb from limb, when we would never do so with a similar congregation of animals. We who are vegetarians seldom demonstrate the same sensitivity with broccoli or soybeans that we do with cows and chickens.

Yet unbeknownst to many, plants are sentient beings, in the full sense of the term. They have senses of sight, smell, hearing, feeling, proportion, and memory, and they process sensory input. They do all this even though they do not have eyes, noses, or other sensory receptors like ours.

Even though there is no apparent similarity in the sensory organs of plants and animals, the gene grouping responsible for the ability of each of them to determine if it is light or dark is the same. Across the board, it turns out that genetic differences between plants and animals are not all that significant.

Animal Guides

When we step onto a Healing Nature Trail, we Walk into the ways of our Native ancestors. Rather than an observational experience, we are immersing ourselves in a living diorama, vibrant with creatures large and small, vocal and silent, flying, crawling, walking, and swimming. Some inhabit the Trail environs, and others are just passing through.

Many of these animals have long served our ancestors as their most trusted guides and life companions. Our species' fascination with the other animals has been the connecting thread of the human lineage across the ages. Many of the earliest known paintings, pendants, and pottery include references to animals. The same is true of the legends, manuscripts, and astronomical symbols we cherish from times past. Nowadays, tattoos, names, icons, and brands continue to draw upon animals for inspiration. The Guardian Angel of the Judeo-Christian tradition is a contemporary parallel that can help us understand the traditional Animal Guide relationship and how it functions on a personal level in daily life.

A commonly used term for the sacred bond between Humans and Animals (and plants) is the "Dodemic relationship." It is our deepest relationship, closer even than our relationship with others of our kind. A Native might consider it to be so intimate that she views herself and her Animal Guide, or *Dodem*, to be of one life. In the fullest sense, the term *Dodem* means *the relationship from which one gains sustenance, sense of self, and meaning in life.* When a Native says, "Cougar is my Dodem," she is essentially saying, "Cougar and I are of the same heart and spirit."

The Dodemic relationship is closely related to the shamanic traditions found in many Native cultures. Around the world, shamanic healers often transform into the animals who give them the power to Journey into the Netherworld to retrieve the lost part of a soul or to bring back a healing formulation or ritual. This is known variously as *Shapeshifting, Animal Transformation, Skin Walking, Otherkinning,* and *Zoanthropy.*

How to Listen

Nearly everyone can recall a special moment when we were in total conscious rapport with another animal. Most of us still find ourselves drawn to animals in many ways and we feel an intrinsic urge to communicate with them.

Yet it is not necessary to know who your Dodem is in order to receive the wisdom and guidance of animals on a Healing Nature Trail. Whether insect or mammal, reptile or bird, amphibian or fish, they are all in regular communication with each other, and they would welcome you to join in on the conversation.

To avail yourself of the full transformative potential of the Trail, it is necessary to attune to what Rumi referred to as the "voice that doesn't use words." Rumi went on to say that all we need in order to understand it is to "listen." Healing Nature Guides are trained to help your listening skills. As well, you can let your intuition guide you. Watch what creatures come your way and which plants draw your attention. Pay particular note to sounds and movements that appear to be just a bit out of the ordinary, as they are often the initial feelers put out by someone who has something to share with you. Note the voices that resonate with you most. Go ahead and reply, in whatever way comes to you—silently, vocally, or with body language.

Voices can come from the strangest of places: a stone, a wilted flower, or even an overhead cloud. Set foot in Nature with an open mind and heart, and there is a good chance you will hear the voices. Be open to plants of all ages, not just the elder trees, as they all have wisdom to share with us.

You can potentially hear from any and all animals and plants. Most of us tend to romanticize—and only listen to—stately trees, charismatic land animals, and great, soaring birds. Yet some of the stories of the beautiful breakthroughs we have heard from Trail users have come from such seemingly unlikely sources as a blade of Grass being chewed on by a Grasshopper, a biting Mosquito, and an Acorn sprouting from a rotting tree stump.

To accompany and empower you on this key component of your Trail Walk, consider taking an *Animal Token* or two along with you. Also known as *Talismans* or *Charms*, Tokens are pocket-size likenesses of Animal Guides that are typically crafted from wood, stone, or clay. Remember to bring your own from home, or to choose one in the outfitting section of the Trail Welcome Center, if it has Tokens available for such use.

If at the end of your Walk you could use some help in interpreting any encounters you had, your Trail Guide is trained to assist. Your therapist may be able to help as well. Some Trails have staff in addition to Trail Guides who are available to consult.

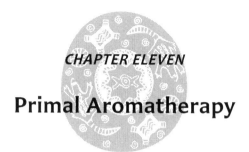

CHAPTER ELEVEN

Primal Aromatherapy

Robert Louis Stevenson said, "It is not so much for its beauty that the forest makes a claim upon men's hearts, as for that subtle something, that quality of the air, that emanation from the old trees, that so wonderfully changes and renews a weary spirit." That "subtle something" can be as minute as a single molecule of an odor that a plant emits, as that's all it takes for the receptor cells in our noses to detect a new smell.

Plants emit these odors to attract animals, which is why one of the first things we usually notice when we leave the city for the great outdoors is the refreshing scent of the air. Stepping into a forest, meadow or wetland opens our noses to a new world of essences. Some change as slowly as the seasons, and others as immediately as one step to the next. Sometimes the smells are totally encompassing, as when the forest is in bloom. At other times the bouquet is subtle, inviting us to bend down and investigate which flower it might emanate from. Or maybe it's the soil itself, so we bend even lower to test our hypothesis.

All of these aromatic curiosities represent one of the most ancient forms of communication. An alluring fragrance attracts a Bee or Butterfly, which carries the pollen from plant to plant that helps them reproduce. Another Insect begins to feast on a leaf, which triggers the plant to release a malodorous repellent.

Ancient Healing Essences

The first sense to evolve in animals was that of smell. Our olfactory nerves help us detect danger, forage for food, and find sexual partners. In addition, our ability to detect certain odors helps us remain healthy and recover from disease. It's based on a complex mode of olfactory communication with the plant world.

Our distant ancestors discovered that certain aromatic plants had positive effects on our physical and psycho-emotional well-being. Thanks to ancient literature and modern archeology, we know that we humans have long been extracting the beneficial compounds from numerous plants, in the form of resins and oils. The practice of using these compounds medicinally and therapeutically is called "Aromatherapy."

Some of these plant-derived compounds were so valued in the era of early civilizations that entire economies were developed around their production and distribution. Frankincense and Myrrh, aromatic resins from trees found in the Middle East, were actively traded along what came to be known as the Incense Road, as they were highly prized what is now Rome, Greece, Egypt, and Israel. The resins were put to many uses: funerary (to mask the stench of decay), medicinal (for nausea relief, post-partum recovery, deterring malaria-infected mosquitos), and spiritual (as an offering to numerous deities).

Aromatherapy is currently used to:

- Strengthen the immune system
- Reduce inflammation
- Encourage the healing process
- Aid decongestion
- Disinfect air and surfaces (antiviral, antibacterial, and anti-fungal)
- Repel biting and other parasitic insects
- Significantly decrease anxiety

- Lower perceived stress and depression
- Improve sleep quality
- Enhance mood
- Improve memory
- Numerous other applications

Preparing for Primal Aromatherapy

When in Nature, we are awash in what is literally the Breath of Life. The effectiveness of that regenerative essence is based entirely on how well we can assimilate it—how well we can make Nature's breath our breath. Breathe slowly through your nose to fully saturate your olfactory receptors.

Exercising your sense of smell enhances the experience of Aromatherapy. Whether you live in a rural or urban environment, indoors or outdoors, make a practice of noticing the variety of smells you encounter. Describe the smells in words and compare them with other familiar smells. Building your vocabulary for smells can help you distinguish nuances amongst even familiar odors.

Unfortunately, some of our modern eating and oral hygiene habits have the effect of dulling our sense of smell. Here are some suggestions for sharpening our olfactory abilities before engaging in Aromatherapy or Walking a Healing Nature Trail. Refrain from:

- Smoking
- Using toothpaste or mouthwash
- Wearing perfume or cologne
- Eating a meal with hot sauce or high salt content

The Trail of Essences

Along a Healing Nature Trail, you have the opportunity to partake in the health benefits offered by a number of aromatic herbs and trees. There may be Wild Mints and Sunflowers, or Willows and Cattails, or Birch and Pine, or Cactus and Sage. Whatever the habitat and composition of the vegetation, there will be numerous members of the plant community continually diffusing their volatile oils into the air.

On many Trails, branches, Ferns, and Grasses are allowed to overhang enough that Walkers brush against them, which stimulates them to release their aromatic essences.

As you Walk, you are likely to experience a peaceful—even euphoric—feeling. The trees and other plants, along with the Wind and running Water, are generating negative ions that clean the air we breathe, boost our immune systems, and lift our moods.

FULL-BODY AROMATHERAPY

Our skin is our largest organ. Among the many ways it serves us is to manufacture nutrients and emit toxins it breathes. These functions are benefited by Aromatherapy, so on the Trail, wear loose clothing and expose as much of your skin to the air as is comfortable for you.

Makwa Giizis, an Ojibwe Elder whom Healing Nature Trail System cofounder Tamarack Song studied under, taught him about the cleansing, centering, and healing energy that comes from hugging trees. He would take people into the forest and have them choose an Elder Tree who spoke to them. Then he would have them hug the tree, breathe into a cleft in the bark, and inhale the infused air the tree gave back. You'll notice benches placed adjacent to elder trees along the Trails specifically for this purpose.

Sunshine, moisture, and moving air are the primary stimulants for plants to release their aromatics. Hug a tree on the side that the sun's rays have warmed, especially after a fresh rain. In lieu of rain, the moisture from your breath has a similar effect.

For a more concentrated dose of a plant's healing essences, crush the needles or leaves by rubbing them between the palms of your hands, cup your hands around your nose, then inhale. Again, do so only under the supervision of a Healing Nature Guide to assure that you have selected a safe and proper species.

CLEANSING YOUR OLFACTORY PALATE

Scents, like the flavors of foods and drinks, can overlap, blend, and numb your olfactory receptors. This diminishes both the pleasurable and medicinal effects of plant essences, a condition known as nasal fatigue. To refresh yourself, move well away from the source of the essence and take several long, full breaths through your nose. Inhale deeply and exhale completely. Another method is to smell your own clean skin.

CHAPTER TWELVE

Talismanic Voices: Drums, Tokens, Feathers, and Crystals

We need other voices to mirror us, challenge us, inspire us. As social creatures, we need the comfort of companionship. We need the synergistic effect that comes from joining with others on the same venture.

Right away we think, "That means I need to involve somebody else in my process." Perhaps. But perhaps not. There is value in working with others of our kind, and there is value in truly detached, other-realm engagement.

Our kind who still live on their Mother's unfettered bosom recognize that all of the components of Nature possess life and spirit. This includes the forces of Nature, such as volcanoes, storms, and earthquakes. It also includes the primary elements of Earth, Air, Fire, and Water, and what comprises them. A Stone, a Feather, a Candle Flame …they breathe and speak, just like you and me.

We know this intuitively, and we practice it when we give someone a farewell gift to take along with them, or when we take a book along with us on a trip. We wear amulets and carry keepsakes for the same reason. Let's look at who we might bring along with us on our Trail Walk. A variety of power objects, representations of Dodems and other animals, and centering tools, will be presented here, so that we can each let our intuitive selves select the traveling companion (or companions) who can best serve us.

The Drum

Life starts and ends with the heartbeat. We breathe to the rhythm of the heart; we love and dance and cry to the rhythm of the heart. The Earth, and the very Cosmos, pulsate with their own heart-rhythm.

All of the sundry hearts know one rhythm—one heartbeat. It is the core of relationship, for when everything else is stripped away we can feel it in everything and everyone. In this most fundamental of ways, we are all related. We all know the same language, we all know the same Way of Being.

When we fall out of sync with the Heartbeat, we get sick. It starts with stress. We feel disjointed, out of touch. Things quit working for us and we struggle in our relationships. Physical ailments crop up and the shadows in the dark reaches of our minds come out to haunt us.

We need to reconnect with the Heartbeat.

The Drum is the way of our kind to rejoin. In the beat of the Drum, we hear the fall of the hoof, the rumble of the storm, and the tremble of the Earth. Drum is the primal musical instrument, the first vehicle beyond voice to express our inner yearnings. Drum is so elemental to the Human experience that she is the only universal instrument. She is the heart of close-to-the-Earth peoples—the center of their social and ceremonial lives. She is so respected in some cultures that all activity stops when she is being played and needs attention.

On the Trail, a Healing Drum is played softly, to let her resonance speak more than her volume. Hold her close to your body or put her on your lap so you can feel the vibration, feel her pulse. Your body then becomes an extension of the Drum—a conveyance of your heartbeat to your Mother Earth, and vice versa. And play the Drum slowly, one beat at a time, until you find the heartbeat of the Drum. On its own, it will then come into sync with your heartbeat, then the Universal Heartbeat, and you will return to Balance.

Our bodies are Drums, which we can play by clapping hands, slapping thighs, stamping feet, or beating chests. Rattles are Drum's younger siblings. Play them in the same way as Drum, slowly to find their heartbeat, then let them find the beat of your heart and bring it into resonance with the Great Heartbeat. Rain-sticks (also known as *Rattle Sticks*) are the most difficult of the elemental rhythm makers to play, and for this reason they can be the most effective.

Tokens

Known also as *Charms, Amulets, Talismans,* and *Fetishes,* Tokens are likenesses of Animal Guides, inscriptions, symbols, or any other representation that exercises a significant influence on a person's feelings or actions. Typically in the form of rings, figurines, and engravings, Tokens are made of malleable materials such as stone, bone, antler, shell, wood, clay, and metal. Some people wear them as pendants, rings, or bracelets, while others carry them in a purse, pack, or pocket.

Indigenous people around the world carve small animal Tokens from the materials listed above. These people consider the Tokens to be alive, in that the spirits of the animals live within them.

Many people like to carry more than one Token, or accompany it with a verse or book excerpt. This works as long as the addition is complementary to the original Talisman. Incompatible or opposing influences can wreak havoc—especially in circumstances like Trail Walks, where the preparation involves relaxing boundaries to become trusting and receptive.

Feathers

Feathers appeal especially to those who have Birds for Animal Guides. Feathers can represent specific Birds or they can generally be valuable for those who see Birds as symbols and metaphors for aspects of their Life Journeys. For some people, Feathers represent

Guardian Angels, who are cultural variations of Animal Guides. For others, Feathers are mementos associated with pivotal times in their lives, or gifts that carry meaning because of the contexts in which they were given.

The size, shape, color, and texture of Feathers create their personalities and hint at the gifts they have to share. Worn and stained Feathers show resilience and steadfastness. Brightly colored and iridescent Feathers are mirrors and magnifiers. Stiff-quilled Feathers encourage inner strength and seeking truth and clarity.

It is suggested that Trail Walkers bring significant Feathers with them. Some welcome centers have Feathers for loan.

Crystals

Nature's primary elements—Earth, Air, Fire, and Water—come together to create her skeleton of Stone. Embedded in the mineral composition and crystalline structure of Stones are the energies of those primary elements. Due to their makeup, some Stones have unique properties that can be called upon to support healing and awakening. These Stones are commonly referred to as *Crystals.*

The vast array of Crystals gives the person drawn to use them seemingly endless choices. Yet, as with Feathers, certain Crystals speak to certain people. Some Crystals appear seemingly by happenstance, and others come as gifts. In addition to their clarifying and regenerative properties, some Crystals hold commemorative meaning.

Crystals of a wide variety of sizes, shapes, and structures figure prominently in the original Healing Nature Trail. The Gateway Labyrinth, Cosmorinth, Cairn, Zen Untangle, and Zen Garden all feature Crystals.

Trail Walkers are reminded to bring Crystals with them that they find helpful. Some Trail welcome centers have a selection of Crystals available for Walkers to choose from and take along with them on the Trail, or to leave at the Cairn at the entryway to the Trail.

Manifesting Your Inner Token

Some of us are verbally oriented, while others have a strong tactile sense. Substantive objects such as Figurines, Feathers, and Crystals tend to work well for us. Yet that may not be the case for those who are visually oriented. They do not always have symbolic mirrors to stand before or traveling companions they can talk easily with like the rest of us. They tend to prefer a way other than words to help convey a deep thought or feeling. The same can apply to journaling, or even to expressing themselves in the moment.

To meet their various needs, some turn to self-rendered images. Many visually oriented people are artists, or at least like to sketch and doodle. They are encouraged to take some favorite art supplies with them on the Trail.

Drawing or sketching can be therapeutic in and of itself, even for those who are not visually oriented. It provides a way to:

 ▶ Strengthen the body-mind connection

 ▶ Navigate the Labyrinthine Mind

 ▶ Release troubled thoughts or repressed feelings

 ▶ Work problems out graphically

 ▶ Envision a new reality

 ▶ Chart a course toward that reality

For deeply wounded individuals, drawing provides a way to access trauma memories that cannot be voiced (or sometimes even recognized) because of fear, conditioning, or denial. However, Trail protocols require that such work be undertaken only under the direct supervision of an authorized therapist.

In the information packets sent out to prospective Trail Walkers, it is suggested that they bring from home any Drums, Rattles, Tokens, Feathers, and Crystals that they would like to use. Some Trail welcome centers have these items available, along with colored pencils, watercolors, crayons, charcoal, and sketch pads.

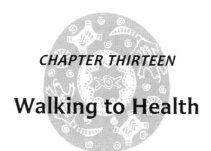

CHAPTER THIRTEEN

Walking to Health

Regular walking is so effective at maintaining centeredness that it could be one of the main reasons people are drawn to Walking Meditation, and to walking in general. At the same time, the quality of an experience is based not only on what we do, but on how we do it. A conscious approach to walking can magnify its benefits.

Urbanized people are typically centered in their heads when they walk. They start each step by moving their heads forward first, which causes them to lean into their steps. They then end up coming down heavily on their heels in order to continually catch themselves.

This plodding-along walking style keeps people head-centered and disconnected from the body. As well, such walking is hard on the feet, leg joints, and lower back, even though it works adequately for getting from point A to point B over prepared surfaces.

In Nature, however, no two steps are the same. In order to move smoothly and quietly—and to keep from tripping—we have to adjust every step to the terrain. And there can be a lot going on between points A and B, so we may need to quickly stop or change direction at any time. That all takes presence, sensory acuity, and functioning from our belly-centers rather than our heads.

We can thank the body-mind connection, as Conscious Walking's clarity of movement strongly encourages clarity of intention. Here's how it's done:

1. **Wear soft-soled shoes** or go barefoot.

2. **Stand up straight,** with knees slightly bent and arms relaxed at your side.

3. **Take a few deep, slow, centering breaths,** all the way down into your belly.

4. **Lift one foot,** as though you are going to take a step, and hold it there while you take another breath.

5. **Step forward,** shortening your stride by about one-third, and coming down on the ball of your foot rather than your heel.

6. **Take another step,** directly in front of the first, as though you were walking on a line.

7. **Proceed slowly,** as though you were stalking up behind someone.

8. **Let your body do the walking** so your head is free to observe, smell, and listen. Glance down only once every few paces to see where you will be stepping.

Some people like to Conscious-Walk the whole Trail. They say it slows them down and keeps them attuned to their surroundings. When they compare with times that they do not Conscious Walk, they realize they notice more, and they feel a deeper sense of satisfaction with their Walk overall.

Healing Nature Guides typically give their clients instruction in Conscious Walking. Following is a general description of the workshop Guides and many Trail organizations offer.

Conscious Walking Workshop

For improving Walking Meditation, Blindfold Walking, and sensory perception, and for training to guide people who are sight-impaired.

Imagine Walking in a special way—with a sense of presence, and with an intent that goes beyond merely reaching a destination. This workshop teaches you how to feel with your feet, and how to use physical movement to create new movement in your mind and heart.

You begin by Walking the Labyrinth, to wind down and get centered. You then get instruction in:

Deerstepping, develops sensitivity by coming down gingerly on the ball of the foot rather than the heel.

Wolf Walking creates a sense of presence through shadowing the person in front of you by stepping in his/her footprints.

Blindfold Walking suppresses sight to supercharge the other senses and stimulate psycho-emotional activity. It includes training for Trail Walkers who are blindfolded or sight-impaired.

Each of the three forms of Walking can be practiced independently; they are taught in sequence, as one prepares for the next. Combining them has a synergistic effect.

The workshop culminates with putting everything to practice on a Healing Nature Trail Walk.

Some Trail organizations offer special Blindfold Walking Workshops for couples, which many find to be a unique and powerful bonding experience.

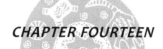

Meditations for the Walk

There are two general types of Healing Nature Trail Walks; those that are intentional, structured, and guided, and those that are unintentional, free-form, and self-guided. People whose relationships are in turmoil, have health crises, or are tormented by inner demons, come to Nature with clear intention. Their sense of purpose supports their Walk in these essential ways:

▶ Energizes them physically and psychically

▶ Keeps them attuned to the Trail experience

▶ Helps them choose which Trail features would best serve them

▶ Gives their Guide clear direction

▶ Makes their overall Walk maximally effective

As valuable as intention can be, it can also blind—especially when one focuses too hard on it. There is the risk of overstimulation and losing perspective. As contradictory and confusing as it might sound, there is a point on the Walk where intention needs to become unintentional.

Intention-Softening Meditations

Here are two meditations that can be practiced at any time on the Trail when intention starts to take over. For the first meditation, repeat the words slowly, with a pause between each phrase. For the second meditation (from Thich Nhat Hahn), inhale and exhale slowly and fully. Do the meditations while Walking, to engage body, mind, and spirit. Some people like to have their Guide recite the meditations, which helps a person fully relax into it.

There is nothing to do
nothing to change
nothing to fix
nothing to heal

(On the inhale) I have arrived.
(On the exhale) I am home.

When Intention Escapes You

Sometimes a person feels troubled, and she's not sure why. Nothing seems to be going right. Her life seems to be no more than a series of dead-end jobs and unfulfilling relationships. A cloud of depression hangs over her. Her spirit screams for change, but she doesn't know what to ask for.

She's gone to a couple of therapists, and she's worked through a number of self-help books. Each was helpful, but each time the effect eventually wore off.

So here she stands at the start of the Trail. What can she do to find clarity of intention?

Fortunately for her, clarity of intention does not necessarily mean having a clear intention, but rather being clear that here is the place—and now is the time—to Walk her Healing Journey. Following are two time-proven ways, one verbal and one nonverbal, to distill that clarity of intention.

An Affirmation

When we verbally state something that we are going to do, we empower and clarify the action. The result then usually better meets our need than it would have had we not verbalized it.

Affirmations serve the purpose well, and here is a favorite that Guides share with their clients:

1. Now is my time to awaken and heal, and I know that Nature's way is my way to do it.

2. I believe in my ability to come together with Nature and co-create joy and healing for myself.

3. I allow myself to believe that I deserve Nature's healing gifts.

4. I give my whole being—body, mind, and spirit—over to becoming a vessel for Nature's healing gifts.

5. With Mother Nature's support, I have the ability to recognize, process, and release all repressed feelings, old stories, and harmful behaviors.

Walking to Intention

There are times when words don't seem to fit. The birds are singing, the breeze is playing in the branches, and we came here to listen. Besides, we don't want to break the personal silence we worked to achieve.

Yet we are losing our clarity of intention. Or maybe we were fooling ourselves by thinking we had it.

We can bring it back with a form of Walking Meditation called *Conscious Walking*. Also known as *Deer Stepping, Fox Walking, and Native Walking*, it is the way Native people move through natural environments in order to keep centered and consciously engaged with their surroundings. You can learn about Conscious Walking in the previous chapter, and you can take a Conscious Walking Workshop at most Healing Nature Trails.

Meditations for No-Intention Walks

From Zen perspective, the idea of setting specific intentions is a grand illusion. How can we know what we need if we have never had it? Or if we think we once did, is it possible that we lost it because we needed something other than that? Something deeper? Or perhaps we already had it and couldn't recognize it?

The more present we are, the less we feel the need to seek. Following are Walking Meditations with no other intention than to be fully present. They were chosen for their simplicity, and for the comfortable doorways they open to the self. Rather than choosing a meditation, let it choose you.

Awakening the Senses

Start by Walking Consciously for fifteen-to-twenty minutes, then become one of your senses for an equal amount of time. Either continue walking or sit/stand in a place that calls to you. The important thing is to fully immerse yourself in the sense you choose, then breathe the experience into your being.

Here is your menu of choices:

Touch
Listen
Smell
Taste
Look

Rewilding

Who you are is who you forgot you were. You can remember by

Slowing down.
Breathing in your surroundings.
Breathing out your thoughts and watching them vaporize.
Lifting your wings to the wind.
Slowing down again.
Becoming your impulses.
Letting your mind dance.
Flowing with the wind and water.
Feeling the lacy treetops.
Slowing down some more.

Zen Meditations

Make a random choice of one of the following meditations, then Consciously Walk with it until it melts away. (See chapter 12 for guidance on Conscious Walking.)

In one falling leaf lives the whole of autumn.

A baby acts without knowing why and moves without knowing where.

Speak rather than answer.

A heavy snowfall disappears into the sea.

I cannot be angry or argumentative with you. It can only be with my illusion of you.

We see things not as they are, but as we are.

If I think something rings true, the opposite also rings true.

By inhaling I show that I am capable of taking in life.

Only from nothing can something arise.

Peace can be found only in death.

The Path becomes the obstacle.

All fear amounts to fear of death.

Truth cannot be written or spoken; it can only be lived.

To assert something is to miss it altogether.

A flower has no meaning unless it blooms.

To admit I am a fool is to find trust in who I am.

Wants and needs are the same.

If I try to keep it, I am already mistaken.

Every moment, I create something.

Cursed rain brings the beautiful mist that filters through the treetops.

CHAPTER FIFTEEN

A Trail for Those with Special Needs

One word captures the focus of all Healing Nature Trail staff—accessibility. They dedicate themselves to making Nature's healing powers accessible to all. This poses unique challenges for the staff to overcome, first because the chasm between Nature and modern humans is already extreme, and second because it can be even more extreme for people with certain physical or psycho-emotional conditions.

Yet, thanks to dedicated individuals and the wonders of human ingenuity, nearly everyone's needs for healing Nature immersion can be met on most Healing Nature Trails. If you have special needs, or if you know or care for someone who does, please do not hesitate to contact a Trail office and see what is possible.

From a Nature-immersion perspective, people with special needs fall into three categories:

▶ Those with physical or psycho-emotional conditions that require specific adaptations.

▶ Those with unique abilities for communing with Nature.

▶ Those who do not have direct access to a Trail, or who are not able to travel.

Let's take a close look at each of these categories, through the lens of how the parent Healing Nature Trail in Wisconsin meets these needs.

Physical and Psycho-Emotional Conditions

This category covers by far the greatest number of people who need special services. In terms of physical conditions, Healing Nature Guides are trained to guide people with limited mobility, those who use wheelchairs or crutches, and people who have sight impairments. Following are the general groupings of people in this category, along with how their Nature-immersion needs can be met.

Limited Mobility

This grouping includes individuals who are able to Walk but have limited ability to do so. The typical reasons for such are cardiovascular conditions, diabetes, obesity, congenital conditions, amputations, age, disease, or recovering from medical procedures. Accommodating Trail features are listed in chapter 27 of the main book, *The Healing Nature Trail*. Standard accommodations provided by the Trail staff at the Welcome Center include:

- Portable fold-up chairs
- Canes with wide pads, to prevent sinking into the ground
- Wide pads for crutches, which must be used on the Woodland Wheels Trail (described under next grouping), due to the narrowness of the Main Trail

Wheelchair and Crutch-Mobile

The main Healing Nature Trail is too narrow and rugged, and many sections have too steep a gradient, to accommodate wheelchairs. For these reasons, the Healing Nature Center has developed a separate Trail system that meets the criteria for wheelchair accessibility.

The Woodland Wheels Trail can accommodate most light- to medium-weight wheelchairs of standard width. The Center Director makes the final determination regarding the suitability of a particular wheelchair for the Trail.

Some Healing Nature Trails have all-terrain wheelchairs for use. They can negotiate steeper gradients and obstacles than typical wheelchairs, and they are less prone to tipping.

Due to the Trail variables, the proximity to water, and fire exposure, Trail users in wheelchairs and on crutches must be accompanied by a specially trained staff member, which includes Healing Nature Guides.

Woodland Wheels Trail features include:

▶ A wheelchair and crutch-accessible Labyrinth

▶ Smudging by being brushed with balsam fir boughs

▶ A wheelchair and crutch-level Cairn

▶ A low-gradient Threshold Bridge

▶ A private Trailside Haven

▶ A specially equipped canoe for the Aquarinth

▶ A Fire-reflection circle and adjacent pond

Sight-Impaired

This grouping includes functionally blind individuals, as well as those vision-compromised to the point that they need a Guide to safely negotiate and have a quality Trail experience. In partnership with the sight-impaired individual, the Center Director helps determine whether or not the individual needs trained assistance for the Trail. Healing Nature Guides are trained to act as Guides for people who are blind.

From a Nature-healing perspective, *sight-impaired* is a misnomer. Most of us rely on sight for 85 percent of our sensory input. Consequently, we miss much of what our other senses could be providing us if we lived in an environmental context where sensory input was more evenly balanced.

Sight-impaired people, on the other hand, benefit from the reverse situation. The acuity of their senses of hearing, smell, taste, and touch is magnified beyond that of sighted people. The same is true of their spatial and movement sensitivities. One could say they are gifted in these areas.

This giftedness gives people who are blind and vision-compromised a unique opportunity to benefit maximally from a number of Trail features and Nature's healing gifts, such as:

▶ Aromatherapy

▶ Grounding

▶ Nature's guiding voices

▶ Conscious Breathing

▶ The body-mind connection, catalyzed by changes in elevation and direction

▶ Bridge sway, particularly on the long, low Bridge that follows the Zen Garden over Troubled Water

▶ Panoramic vistas, experienced by stereoscopic sound, the feel of the breeze, and the touch of the sun

▶ The Labyrinth of Sound, comprised of the variety and complexity of Nature's voices

▶ Finger Labyrinths

▶ The Zen Garden

▶ The sound of the Drum, Rattle, and Rainstick (available at the Welcome Center for Trail use)

▶ The feel of a Token (also available at the Welcome Center)

Psycho-Emotional Conditions

Healing Nature Guides are trained to work with the therapists or guardians of many individuals with psycho-emotional conditions that inhibit their ability to independently Walk the Trail. The Center Director has the ultimate authority to determine an individual's capability for negotiating the Trail, whether or not that individual is accompanied by a healthcare practitioner, guardian, or Guide. The Center Director works in collaboration with the individual Walker and his or her therapist to make that decision.

Unique Abilities

As with the sight-impaired, many individuals diagnosed with conditions such as autism, hypersensitivity, ADD/ADHD, and depression, or who are symptomatic of such conditions, find that some of their symptoms become assets on the Trail. Some autistic people have a knack for understanding the language of animals, hypersensitive individuals sometimes respond quickly to Aromatherapy, and those with attention-deficit traits often notice more than others.

Some individuals in this grouping are best served by Trail Walks modified to meet their particular needs and abilities. These determinations are made by the individual's therapist in consultation with the Trail Guide working with them, or with the Center Director.

Another grouping under this banner includes those with unique or exceptional physical abilities, such as tree climbing, swimming, running, or tracking, which can serve as catalysts for a heightened Trail experience. Trail Guides are trained to help design Walks that incorporate these aptitudes to take full advantage of the healing and awakening opportunities a Trail Walk affords.

For example, what can be provided for tree climbers is Treetop Breathing in Nature, Aromatherapy, Panoramic Vistas, and Labyrinthine Envisioning. These climbing experiences are facilitated by Healing Nature Guides who are Certified Recreational Tree Climbing Instructors.

Inability to Access a Trail

Some physical and psychological conditions keep people either bedbound or housebound. For various reasons, a number of others are unable to travel to a Healing Nature Trail. Fortunately, this book and related online resources can bring the Trail to them, by way of a process called *Remote Walking*.

The founders and directors devoted considerable energy toward making Remote Walking a key feature of the Healing

Nature Trail concept. They wanted the restorative properties of Nature to be available to everyone, including people who are immobile.

Remote Walking also benefits those who are physically challenged and cannot Walk the complete Trail or take advantage of all the Trail has to offer. Someone with impaired breathing can then still be helped by Aromatherapy, and someone who cannot negotiate the Zen Untangle or Aquarinth can yet experience them and gain from them.

Why Remote Walking Is Possible

Recent research shows that many of the benefits of Nature Immersion can be attained by merely viewing Nature through a window. Even more remarkably, a similar effect can be gained by gazing at an online photo or a mural of a Nature scene.

The reason a view or image of Nature works is that they help us imagine we are immersed in Nature. The ability to do so is called *Envisioning*. All animals, including humans, generally relate to their environment through their senses. We rely on smell, sight, hearing, and touch to find food and shelter, and to navigate.

In addition, we can Envision, and as far as we know, we are the only animals capable of doing so. Here's how Envisioning works: If we were hunting an animal, we could create a mental picture of where to find her, based on our knowledge of the animal's habits and habitat. This saves us the laborious — and often unsuccessful — task of directly following the footprints or scent of our prey over long distances in order to catch up with it, as other animals have to do.

Envisioning, then, gives us the ability to perform beyond the capabilities of our physical senses. We are able to mentally create what does not exist, and what exists beyond the reach of our senses. *Once we create it, we can experience and gain from it.*

How Remote Walking Is Accomplished

In her ultimate wisdom, Mother Nature provided us with the quintessential place for our minds to open and our spirits to soar. The Trail developers are the first to admit that it was not them, but Nature, who designed the Trail. They merely listened to her guidance. We can do the same through Remote Walking; we can close our eyes and Envision, and the Trail will appear in the landscape of our minds. We can then set foot upon it.

Here's how it is done:

1. Find a quiet place, free of distractions.

2. Center yourself by taking several slow, deep breaths.

3. Invite your personal Guide to join you by opening this book to Part I: *Walking the Trail,* and playing a recording of Northwoods Nature sounds.

   or

4. Watch *A Walk on the Wild Side,* a video-recorded Trail Walk.

5. Envision being there: the wind swaying the Trees, Chipmunks scampering about, an Eagle soaring overhead, and people like you Walking the Labyrinth and Trail.

6. Take your shoes off, step on a soft rug, and imagine you're feeling the mossy ground underfoot.

7. Walk your fingertip along the Path of a Finger Labyrinth (or paper image of a Labyrinth) while reading or viewing the Labyrinthine Walk.

8. Smell the Pine-scented air by placing a few of drops of Aromatherapy Oil on a napkin or in a diffuser.

9. Bathe in a Panoramic Vista by opening your window to let the sun and breeze splash your face.

Guided Remote Walking

There is one more key component of a Trail Walk that you can incorporate into your Remote Walking: a Healing Nature Guide.

The experience and personal stories that a Guide can contribute will bring a Remote Trail Walk all the more to life. Guides have dedicated their lives to doing all they can for Nature-assisted healing, so many of them are willing to travel to a client's home or recovery room, andwould consider it an honor to do so. They can also guide Remote Walkings by telephone and Skype.

As trained storytellers, Guides can take clients on Remote Trail Walks in three different ways:

- ▶ **Reading** a story of a Trail Walk, with pictures, based on Part I of this book.

- ▶ **Narration** accompanying the *A Walk on the Wild Side* video.

- ▶ **Customized Guided Visualization,** to meet a client's personal needs.

To help bring Remote Walks to life, Guides bring with them a photo album, a Finger Labyrinth, smudging boughs, Aromatherapy Oil, some forest soil, and water from the Aquarinth.

Experience shows that a Guide can contribute significantly to the quality and effectiveness of a Remote Walk. For those who are going to be immobilized for extended periods of time, it is quite advantageous for a Guide to facilitate at least the first Remote Walk. The Guide can then train the client to maximize his subsequent self-guided Remote Walk.

BRINGING THE ACTUAL TRAIL TO THE CLIENT

Some Healing Nature Guides have filmed Trail Walks with head-cameras, which allows immobile people to visually take actual Trail Walks, conducted by their personal Guides. Other Guides have the capacity to livestream Walks, which gives Guides and clients the ability to have interactive Trail experiences in real time.

Self-Guided Remote Walking

Here is a simplified Envisioned Trail Walk that you can take on your own anytime, anyplace, with no audio-visual aids needed.

Use it when traveling, lying awake at night, or taking a break at work.

Start with Conscious Breathing (see chapter 8) to bring yourself into the moment and relax into the experience. Then slowly read the following visualization (or have it read to you).

I imagine that I am crossing the Threshold Bridge to enter the Maze known as the Healing Nature Trail. Just before the Bridge, I calmed and centered myself by Walking the Labyrinth. Then on the way to the Bridge, I got brushed by the Pine boughs that hung over the Trail. The aromatic essences they released gave me a cleansing, uplifting Smudge.

Right after that, I came upon the Cairn where I placed the special stone I brought to commemorate my experience.

Now I am about to step off of the archway between two worlds—I have left my travails behind and I am entering the rejuvenating Realm of Nature. Already I feel lighter as I take a deep breath of the clean, Pine-laced Forest air. The comfortingly soft ground beneath my feet makes me feel welcomed as the Trail takes me into a grove of towering Pines.

I feel safe under the protective canopy.

A Tree calls to me and I sit back-to-back with her. I feel her energy coming up from the ground and running along my spine. Closing my eyes, I breathe with the tree. She exhales, and I inhale her breath. I exhale, and she inhales my breath. We are one breath, one life.

Now I hear the wind whistling through the high branches. The Tree responds, listing ever so slightly one way, then the other. Yet I feel it, and I raise my arms to catch the breeze and join in the leisurely dance.

As I sway, my breathing falls in sync with the waves of wind and the swaying tree.

A sigh springs forth spontaneously from me, then a humming sound that harmonizes with the whistle of the wind and the titter of the birds.

I get caught up in the chorus and I want to keep dancing. Yet the Trail beckons. I feel so light that it's as though I'm drifting over the Pathway on the wings of a Butterfly. Am I just high on the fresh, oxygenated air? Or maybe it's the negative ions and endorphins from the trees?

Whatever the case, I feel more alive than I have in a long time. I'm stepping as light as a child, and I'm starting to see through the haze. What a beautiful day it is!

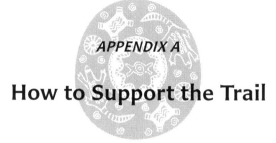

APPENDIX A

How to Support the Trail

The best way to provide and care for the Trail is to use it. The sole reason for its being is to be there for you, so come whenever you feel called. You are always welcome.

As well, you can bring the Trail to others like you by envisioning them Walking the Trail. So many people have lost connection with the Earth and their Path in life. Many more struggle physically and psycho-emotionally. Picture them on the Trail reconnecting with Nature and being bathed in her healing support, and your envisionment will help it happen.

Other ways to support the Trail's reason for being are to **Bring a friend** with you on your next Walk, **Give a Gift Certificate** for a Walk, and **Spread the word** to people you know and work with, including healthcare professionals. You could **post on social media** and **write letters** to the editors of papers and magazines.

The Welcome Center has several possibilities for spreading the word. You can acquire additional copies of either *A Forest Bathing Companion* or *The Healing Nature Trail* to give to others you think would like to know about the Trail. Wearing a Trail T-shirt or hoodie can give a lot of exposure. And if you take a Finger Labyrinth home with you, it is bound to be a conversation piece that leads to your Trail story.

It's All about Relationship

From a Zen perspective, life is relationship, and that's the essence of the Trail experience. Whether it's with Nature, our inner selves, or our fellow Trail lovers, seeking fulfillment in relationships may well be our prime motivator. In this sense, your presence means more than anything when it comes to supporting the Trail.

Following are three special ways your presence can be felt—special because they engender relationship.

Volunteer

There is a wide variety of opportunity for helping to caretake a Healing Nature Trail, both directly and indirectly. Hands-on opportunities include Trail and Labyrinth maintenance, wild-flower gardening, and Bridge and Center repairs (which could include general labor, carpentry, electrical, or plumbing). Sometimes assistance can be used at workshops and other events.

THE LABYRINTHIANS
One volunteering example at the original Healing Nature Trail is a group who call themselves The Labyrinthians. They support the Trail by caring for the Gateway Labyrinth's wildflower beds and trimming the grass.

There always seems to be room for more outreach, whether it's distributing handouts and posters, webpage updating, or writing/editing. Help is often welcomed for fundraisers and grant writing. With any other talent or interest you have, please contact the Director to see how you can be of service.

Join Friends of the Trail

The camaraderie is contagious in the Friends of the Trail group, as its members share a love of Nature and a dedication to making the Healing Nature Trail the best possible gateway to Nature's healing gifts. Regular volunteers, stakeholders, and contributors are invited to join the Friends. Benefits include:

> ❱ Unlimited usage of the Trail for members and their families,

⬧ Invitation to special events held just for the Friends, including an annual banquet,

⬧ Discounts on Healing Nature Center workshops, courses, trainings, and goods.

Be a Trail Development Ambassador

One Healing Nature Trail can serve only so many people and, practically speaking, it is a regional resource. The goal of the Healing Nature Center is to help establish regional Trails across America, Europe, Australia, and wherever else Nature can reach out to her lost and besieged children. This includes Trails accessing us to all of Nature's many spangled forms—prairie, wetland, beach, mountain, desert, rain forest, and taiga.

If you know of an individual or organization who might like to establish a Healing Nature Trail, please ask them to go to www. healingnaturecenter.org, or give them a copy of this book and its companion book, *The Healing Nature Trail,* which gives detailed guidance on how to organize, design, and conduct outreach for a Healing Nature Trail.

Ways to Contribute

This chapter section serves as a guide for financial supporters of the original Healing Nature Trail, and a template for other Trails to develop contribution formats.

Trail usage donations and tuition cover most of the day-to-day Trail and Center overhead. Special services such as the wheelchair-accessible Trail are supported largely by grants. Yet funding is needed on a sustainable basis for Trail development, workshop presentations, expansion of services, outreach, maintenance, wages, and property taxes.

The Trail staff and Friends of the Trail respectfully ask that you consider making a one-time or periodic contribution to support and assure the future of the Trail. This could take the form of donating to the Trail Maintenance Fund, establishing a Memorial, contributing to the Legacy Fund, remembering the Trail in your will, or a monthly contribution charged to your credit card. You may also donate a used vehicle, real estate, artwork, or collectibles. All contributions, monetary or otherwise, are 100 percent tax-deductible.

Following are the various ways you can contribute:

Trail Maintenance Fund

Any amount is accepted. The fund supports the upkeep of the Trail, Labyrinths, and adjacent grounds.

Tokens of appreciation for Trail Maintenance Fund contributions are awarded as follows:

- For all donors of $25 or more—A copy of *The Healing Nature Trail*.
- For donors of $100—A copy of *Becoming Nature* or *Wild Sounds of the Northwoods*.
- For donors of $300—Copies of *Zen Rising* and *Song of Trusting the Heart*.
- For donors of $500—A one-year pass to the Healing Nature Trail.
- For donors of $1000—A Finger Labyrinth (choose from three classic designs) and a one-year Trail pass.
- For donors of $5000—A custom-crafted Finger Labyrinth replica of the Gateway Labyrinth.

In addition, all donors of $1000 or more are recognized with a brass nameplate on a permanent Birchwood Plaque in the Welcome Center. Donors of $5000 or more are specially recognized on the Plaque.

Memorial/Dedication Plaques

$500 for the Trail Bench or Bicycle Rack Plaque.

$750 for the Stump Labyrinth Plaque.

$1000 for the Pollinator Wildflower Bed Plaque.

$2000 for the Hermitage Cabin Plaque.

$3000 for the Zen Untangle or Zen Garden Plaque.

$4000 for the Welcome Center Plaque.

$5000 for the Trance Dance Studio Plaque.

$7500 for the Cosmorinth Plaque.

$10,000 for the Gateway Labyrinth Plaque.

$15,000 for the Threshold Bridge or Trail History Museum Plaque.

The Legacy Fund

The ability of the Healing Nature Center to continue its healing mission well into the future is secured by sustaining contributions from individuals, families, trust funds, and organizations. These contributors provide a support base that makes it possible for the Center to offer the best possible Trail and workshop experiences, along with making the Trail and other Center offerings available to everyone seeking Nature's solace and healing touch, regardless of financial state. Contributions in the form of currency, real estate, bequests, stocks, bonds, and annuities are accepted.

- A $25,000 bequest is honored by a Board of Directors proclamation to install a commemorative sign at the head of the Healing Nature Trail, dedicating it to the memory of whomever the bequester desires.

- A $50,000 bequest is honored by a Board proclamation to mount a commemorative tile beside the door of the Healing Nature Center, dedicating it to the memory of whomever the bequester desires.

- A $100,000 bequest is honored by a Board proclamation to mount a commemorative tile beside the door of the Giant Pine Meeting Lodge, dedicating it to the memory of whomever the bequester desires.

The Trail's Healing Nature Center Family

Comprised of a Nature preserve and a complex of footpaths, Labyrinths, and workshop-retreat spaces, the Healing Nature Center is a 501(c)(3) nonprofit organization charged with the mission to make the therapeutic properties of Nature accessible to individuals, groups, healthcare practitioners, and their clients.

The Center's approach is to create a synergistic format by incorporating shamanic and Zen practices, along with techniques based on contemporary neuroscience and epigenetics research. Primary areas of focus are trauma, stress and anxiety, relationship, self-discovery, reconnecting with Nature, and physical healing support.

As mentioned in the previous chapter, the Center is dedicated to supporting the establishment of regional Healing Nature Trails wherever they can serve people who could benefit from Nature's healing embrace.

The Center's flagship tool is the Healing Nature Trail, a first-of-its-kind Nature-immersion experience that enhances the body-mind connection with somatic sensitizing exercises, Aromatherapy, plant and animal communication, and the shamanic use of breath, Earth, Fire, and Water.

Brother Wolf Foundation

Along with the Trail, the Center sponsors the Brother Wolf Foundation, a long-term project to establish a sanctuary for unwanted domesticated Wolves who cannot be reintroduced into the wilds. In conjunction with the sanctuary, an educational center is going to be established to renew awareness of the ancient Wolf-Human relationship. According to the legends of the Ojibwe people of the Upper Great Lakes region, this kinship has existed since the dawn of creation. It is so close that the destinies of both species are inextricably intertwined. "As goes the fate and fortune of Wolf, so goes the fate and fortune of Man," says one of the Ojibwe legends. This profound relationship is a metaphor for our kinship with all of life.

Environmental Stewardship

The Center runs on the reduce-reuse-recycle philosophy. As much as possible, the Center refrains from buying anything new and sources materials and supplies locally. Old buildings are restored with local salvaged materials, rather than being demolished and replaced.

The Healing Nature Trail features were constructed entirely from salvaged materials. Old docks were turned into walkways, utility poles became bridge pilings, sawmill sawdust was used in Trail paving, and castaway quarry stone became Path borders.

Center staff are active in regional environmental activities, from chairing the Natural Resources Committee to working with local agencies and citizens to eradicate invasive plant species and establish backyard wildlife habitat.

The Campus

Two buildings stand on campus: the Center, which houses the office, bookstore, Trail History Museum, and workshop space; and the Giant Pine Lodge, which offers additional workshop space, along with rooming and eating facilities for Trail Walkers, workshop participants, and presenters.

Rounding out the campus are a Turf Labyrinth and a wheelchair-accessible Labyrinth, two Healing Nature Trails (one is wheelchair accessible), and wildflower beds designed to support dwindling populations of pollinator species such as Bees and Butterflies.

Campus facilities are available for lease to therapists, workshop presenters, and educational and environmental organizations in alignment with the Center's mission.

Center facilities are available for:

- Individuals, groups, and Healing Nature Guides and therapists accompanying their clients to use the Healing Nature Trail
- Labyrinth Walkers
- Meditators (Walking, Sitting, and Paddling)
- Personal and group retreats
- Trainings, courses, and workshops presented by Center faculty and visiting instructors

The Healing Nature Center is a sister organization to Snow Wolf Publishing and Teaching Drum Outdoor School.

The Programs

Consulting

- **Healing Nature Trail Development**. From site selection and design to organization and outreach.
- **Environmental Restoration.** Landscaping and recovery designs for Northwoods habitats, focusing on ecosystem integrity and endangered/invasive species.

Certification and Diploma Programs

- **Healing Nature Trail** certification
- **Associate, Senior, and Off-Trail Healing Nature Guide** diploma courses
- **Suicide Prevention** training and certification

Therapy

- **Trauma Therapy** and management workshops
- **Shamanic Therapy** and training
- **Therapeutic Breathwork** sessions and training
- **Trance Dance** for stress release and deep trauma work

Personal Growth

- **Solo and Group Retreats.**
- **Zen Retreats**
- **Wild Childrearing Training**
- **Animal Guide Workshops**
- **Dreamwork**

Environmental

- **For the Birds, Bees, and Butterflies.** Workshops and tours for school groups, clubs, educators, farmers, and the general public, on establishing high nectar-producing wildflower beds.
- **Wetland Restoration.** The Center is engaged in a model project to restore nine ponds and a stream back to their natural state in the preserve on which it is located.

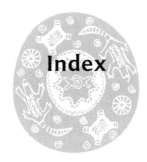

Index

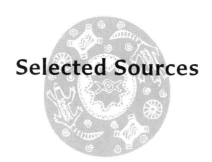

Selected Sources

As previously mentioned, *The Forest Bathing Companion* was created from material in *The Healing Nature Trail: Forest Bathing for Recovery and Awakening* by Tamarack Song. That book's endnotes give a complete accounting of the source material for both books. In addition, *The Healing Nature Trail* includes a comprehensive overview of the healing power of Nature, an introduction to Healing Nature Trails and their history, a workbook for establishing Healing Nature Trails, and a description of Trail certification and Trail Guide degree programs.

Following are resources chosen for those who wish to further explore the main themes presented in this book. Most of the titles are available for purchase at Trail welcome centers.

Becoming Nature: Learning the Language of Wild Animals and Plants by Tamarack Song (Bear & Company, 2016)

Break Through with Breathwork: Jumpstarting Personal Growth in Counseling and the Healing Arts by Jim Morningstar, PhD (North Atlantic Books, 2017)

Cairns: Messengers in Stone by David B. Williams (The Mountaineers Books, 2012)

Classical Labyrinths: Construction Manual by Robert Feere (Labyrinth Enterprises, 2001)

Conscious Breathing: Breathwork for Health, Stress Release, and Personal Mastery by Gay Hendricks, PhD (Bantam Books, 1995)

Entering the Mind of the Tracker: Native Practices for Developing Intuitive Consciousness and Discovering Hidden Nature by Tamarack Song (Bear & Company, 2013)

Last Child in the Woods: Saving Our Children from Nature Deficit Disorder by Richard Louv (Algonquin Books, 2008)

Mazes & Labyrinths: Their History & Development by W. H. Matthews (Dover Publications, 2003)

A Sand County Almanac: with Essays on Conservation from Round River by Aldo Leopold (Ballantine, 1986)

What a Plant Knows: A Field Guide to the Senses by Daniel Chamovitz (Farrar, Straus and Giroux, 2012)

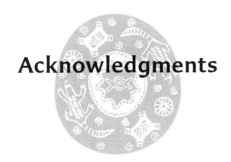

Acknowledgments

I have written a number of books, but not one with near this many contributors. If the front cover was large enough, I would list all of their names along with mine. Yet honoring them here instead has a beautiful advantage—I have the space to acknowledge their contributions as well as them.

Jim Arneson of JAAD Book Design crafted the cover and interior; Amber Braun provided the Gateway Labyrinth design and researched Labyrinth history; Nan Casper transcribed most of the text and provided valuable editorial input; Baerbel Ehrig gave an overview of pollinator bee and butterfly habitat restoration. Michael Fox was the moving force behind building the Trail. He helped design the Trail's features, headed up the construction crew, and did most of the finer work himself. In addition, he researched Cairns and rendered the Trail maps for this book. Without him, the Trail might still be but a dream. Susan Gilman offered her experience in Grounding; Jim Morningstar, PhD, and Steve Moe, LMT contributed to the sections on conscious breathing and the psychology of movement; Michael Patterson shared material on Healing Trails, Zen Gardens, and Labyrinths; Brittany Servent researched academic source material; Claire Sweeney interviewed people on Forest Therapy; Sami True offered her knowledge of Aromatherapy; and a person who wishes to remain anonymous researched Nature-based healing and designed our logo.

Working beside me on nearly every phase of this project was my long-time collaborator and editor, Andrew Huff. Both he and

Stephanie Phibbs, PhD, gave the manuscript a solid proofread, and Pat and Stephanie Morris did the final proof. Brett Schwartz numbered the index and adapted text excerpts from the mother book, *The Healing Nature Trail*.

Even with the strong and fruitful partnership that coalesced, writing this Healing Trail presentation turned out to be a largely solo venture. I needed quiet space and uninterrupted time, which was provided by friends and neighbors Luke and Myriam Brault, and the Edward U. Demmer Memorial Library of Three Lakes, Wisconsin.

Prior to this book project, I did not own a laptop computer and I needed one for my remote writing venues. Early one afternoon, a delivery service brought a brand-new laptop to my doorstep, straight from the manufacturer. To this day I do not know the responsible party.

To each and every one of these valued friends, collaborators, and phantom supporters, I extend my deepest gratitude. Without them, I'd still be lost in some fuzzy dream about what could be and how to achieve it.

Then again, there is one person who would never leave me floating around in my fantasies, pleasant as that might be. My bosom friend, loving mate, and creative partner, Lety Seibel, was an integral part of every phase of not only this book's creation, but also the birthing of the wondrous woodland Trail that this book attempts to reflect. It is here that words must stop, as I have no way other than cherishing her every breath and movement to convey what her all-embracing presence means to me.

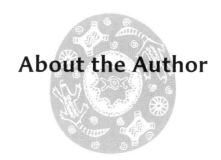

About the Author

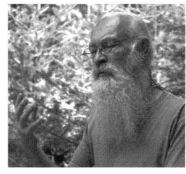

Tamarack Song learned about the healing powers of Nature through academic study, apprenticing to Native shamans and herbalists, living with a pack of wolves, and residing in the wilds for most of his life. He currently lives in the Nicolet National Forest, where he keeps in touch with the wolves and other medicine animals and plants with whom he works.

Tamarack serves as executive director of the Healing Nature Center and he cofounded Healing Nature Trails. He has academic training in stress management, ethics, therapeutic breathwork, conservation, and nonprofit corporation management. His book, *A Forest Bathing Companion*, is based on his Nature-based Healing and Trauma Recovery PhD dissertations. The author of books on shamanic trance healing, suicide prevention, spirit animal guides, animal tracking, Truthspeaking, Native-inspired childrearing, and Zen, he also serves as an environmental restoration and outdoor expedition consultant.

As founder of the Teaching Drum Outdoor School, he has developed management strategies for the psycho-emotional challenges unique to wilderness experiences. He has taught conflict resolution and indigenous living skills, herbalism, and dream therapy for forty years.

58707734R00109

Made in the USA
Columbia, SC
25 May 2019